Harmony in Nutrition

Uniting the Best of Diets

J.B. Craft

Table of Contents

Introduction

Meg was a well-known professional dietician in her community in Chicago. One day, she invited different people who wanted to go on a diet so that everyone understood what pushes people to change the way they eat. It was a Saturday afternoon and Meg had invited five people who were all seated around the table in her boardroom. After introducing herself to her guests, she gave all of her guests a chance to introduce themselves and tell the gathering why they decided to go on a diet. Amongst the guests were Christina, Ronnie, John, Theresa, and Jaiden. Meg was the sixth.

The first person to introduce herself was Theresa who worked as a secretary. She told Meg and the other guests that she had been diagnosed with breast cancer; and besides being on chemotherapy, she was supposed to follow a strict cancer diet. Ronnie was a shopkeeper at a local store who said he could not cope with his weight gain. He told others that his love for food had just become uncontrollable and he now wants to reduce his body weight.

Jaiden said he struggles with indigestion. Every time he eats, he has an upset stomach and the food that he eats takes a long time to digest. John was diagnosed with type 2 diabetes and wished to eat a diet that helps him to control his blood sugar levels. Finally, it was Christina, a model who wanted to lose weight so that she fit well in her career.

Meg then stood up and told her guests that she was happy to hear all the different reasons that her visitors were giving her. She told them that she had seen so many people who wanted to go on a diet because of different reasons. Some are diabetics, some need to eat a diet that is suitable for expecting mothers, and certain individuals want to attain a body that makes them feel more comfortable in their own skin.

Besides the issues that have been mentioned above, there are so many benefits of going on a diet that can include:

- **Lower blood pressure:** When you lose weight, this can also help you to reduce your blood pressure. Losing a bigger percentage of your weight can be very beneficial, but even losing 2 to 5% can help you improve systolic blood pressure.

- **Improving your cholesterol ratio:** Weight loss can also help you increase your good cholesterol or high-density lipoprotein.

- **Reduced risk of heart disease:** When you have reduced high blood pressure as well as lower cholesterol levels, this can also help reduce the risk of heart disease.

- **Reduce your blood glucose levels:** Reduced weight can also make it easier for people with diabetes to control this disease.

- **Good mood:** Besides weight loss and making you look good, it can also help to improve your mood.

- **Improved energy levels:** People who have lost weight also experience higher energy levels. This energy can help improve your exercises and further maintain your required weight.

Now that you understand the benefits of going on a diet, let's go into the first chapter and look at the importance of diets for your health and your overall well-being.

Chapter 1:

Introduction to Diets

What is the meaning of the word "diet"? We can have two definitions for the word. Firstly, the word "diet" can be described as the food and drink that is eaten or consumed by a person or a group of people. The second definition refers to a diet as a specific or controlled consumption of food and drink that is restricted to suit certain needs or for a particular purpose—for instance, a diet for weight loss.

Nutritionally, a supplementary diet can refer to food and drink that is consumed by an individual for a specific health disorder during a particular therapy. The diet must fulfill or meet the nutritional requirements of that individual. Let's take, for example, a person suffering from diabetes who would require food that helps them regulate their blood sugar levels. The diet should consist mainly of fruits and vegetables that contain a lot of dietary fiber.

Human beings are known for consuming an omnivorous diet, but this varies with individual preferences for certain individuals who are selective and refuse to touch other foods, but rely on specific types of food. This is how different kinds of diets were formed, each of them depending on the type of food that is consumed. Below is a list of various kinds of diet:

- The Keto diet

- The DASH diet

- The Plant-based diet

- The Paleo diet

- Intermittent fasting

- Mediterranean diet

- Well balanced diet

- The Vegetarian diet

- The Omnivorous diet

- The Vegan diet

- The Fruitarian diet

- The High Fiber diet

- The Alkaline-ash diet

- The Elimination diet

- The Challenge diet

- The Wilder's diet

Why Diet Is Crucial in Health and Wellness

When we talk of a healthy diet, we are looking at the combination of foods and drinks that will be able to provide you with energy, make you feel great, improve your health, and, at the same time, put you in a good mood. For you to be able to have good health and mental peace, you need to improve your physical activities, get healthy nutrition, and attain an appropriate body weight.

For a diet to be considered a healthy one, it must consist of the right amounts of protein, fats or oils, carbohydrates or starches, mineral elements, and vitamins. Consuming the right amount of calories can help your body to function appropriately, therefore, you need to eat whole grain foods, different types of fruits and vegetables, and a selection of healthy fats and protein. These nutrients are essential to the proper functioning of your body, physically, mentally, and for your overall well-being.

The word essential means that your body cannot function well without these nutrients since they are vital for your growth, as well as developing and maintaining the body's functions. When the nutrient supply to your body does not meet the requirements or the amount needed by the cell activity, this may lead to the slowing down of your metabolic processes. Food nutrients can however be considered as the body's guidance or a source of knowledge on how it performs. This makes us understand and concentrate more on the types of food that we need to consume, instead of what we must not consume.

You have to view food as a vital tool to promote a healthy body, preventing diseases, and improving your overall well-being. You don't have to look at food as something bad. The reason why people end up looking at some foods as the cause of certain disorders like cancer, diabetes, heart disease, or obesity is due to the belief that they are caused by a single gene mutation. However, such diseases are caused by a network of biological dysfunction. The food that you eat can, therefore, play a part in the formation of these conditions because there will be a lack of nutritional balance.

The most important thing for humans to do is to look at the way different types of nutrients interact and impact an individual's body functions in order to stay away from the onsets of these health conditions. You can benefit more from functional medicine, which is the assessment, prevention, and management of chronic illness and complex diseases through the use of a healthy, well-balanced diet.

Let's have a look at how food affects our health. Food provides us with the knowledge and nutrients that our bodies require to work properly. When we don't eat the foods that provide us with all the required nutrients, in correct proportions, our bodies suffer and this results in deteriorating health. We are most likely to suffer from being overweight, or undernourished if we consume too much or too little food.

Eating a well-balanced diet can help our bodies to get nutrients from all the main food classes like fruits and vegetables, whole grains, and lean proteins, as well as healthy fats. When making a choice of your food, make sure you substitute foods that contain added sugar, salt, and trans fats with nutritious foods. Healthy eating can enhance bone strength, improve your mood, and reduce the likelihood of complex diseases.

Hypertension and heart-related illnesses are a big concern in the United States. It is the leading reason for adult deaths in the country. Most adults can suffer heart failure, heart attack, or stroke, which are all conditions related to hypertension and blood pressure. Regular exercise and a well-balanced diet can greatly reduce premature diagnosis of heart disease and stroke.

The recommended diet should include the consumption of multi-colored fruits and vegetables, whole grain foods, low-fat or fat-free dairy products, and meat substitutes like beans, fish, and nuts. Make sure you don't eat foods containing saturated fats. Also, cut down on sugar-sweetened foods and beverages, and reduce sodium intake to less than 2300 mg per day (NIH, 2021). It's also advised to increase the consumption of calcium, magnesium, and potassium.

The consumption of food that is high in fiber can help reduce the risk of heart disease and type 2 diabetes. To lower the levels of cholesterol and lipoprotein, stay away from the consumption of trans fats. This type of fat can cause plaque to form in the arteries which increases the risk of heart issues. You can also reduce your blood pressure by decreasing the amount of salt that you eat per day. Fast foods contain high sodium and should be avoided.

To avoid diseases like cancer, eat more foods that are rich in antioxidants that can prevent cell damage. Free radicals in your body can increase the risk of cancer, but antioxidants can help eliminate these free radicals.

Introduction to the Most Popular Diets in America

No matter what you want to achieve by following a specific diet, the starting point is to change your current eating habits. This process of shifting from one type of diet to another may seem easier said than done. We used to hear experts advising people to simply go on a low-calorie diet, however, in this day and age, the way you view healthy eating may differ from how the person next to you understands it, with fad diets making the confusion worse.

Knowing what is required of you rather than generalizing things is of tantamount importance. Do you have to take into consideration your blood type, or should you go on a low-fat diet? Should you completely take out a certain class of food? At the end of the day, no answer is suitable for every person. The answer to your own diet can be as unique as your fingerprint.

Different Types of Diets

So many diets exist out there, with some giving specific types of foods to consume, while others allow you a variety of foods. The following is a list of the six diets that are currently popular: the Mediterranean diet, intermittent fasting, the keto diet, the DASH diet, the plant-based diet, and the paleo diet. We are going to look at each type of diet in the following chapters.

In this chapter, we concentrated on the importance of a diet for health benefits and our overall well-being. We have also looked at different types of diets that are available for your choice. In the next chapter, we are going to look at the Mediterranean diet in detail including its pros and cons. We will also cover the kind of foods that this type of diet focuses on. Let's dive into Chapter 2 and read more.

The Mediterranean Diet

I am of the opinion that some of the food that we put in our bodies really causes harm to us. It's been seen that people who consume Mediterranean and Japanese diets survive for a very long period. —Cote de Pablo

In Chapter 1, we already covered why a healthy diet is important for our health and a list of different kinds of diets that we have. This chapter is going to cover the Mediterranean diet in full, we will also look at the advantages and disadvantages of using this type of diet.

The Mediterranean diet has recently been ranked as the number one diet in the United States (Carol, 2019). This type of diet is considered to be more of an eating plan rather than a diet schedule. It was discovered that humans who lived within the Mediterranean area survived for longer and had lower rates of suffering from heart disease, cancer, and type 2 diabetes than the way these conditions are affecting Americans. This was found to be a result of their active lifestyle and the type of food that they consume, which consists of less processed foods and more plant-based foods.

What Is the Mediterranean Diet?

The Mediterranean diet can be described as an eating plan that focuses on consuming mainly fruits, vegetables, whole grains, beans, olive oil, herbs, nuts, legumes, and spices. This diet only includes smaller quantities of other foods such as animal protein, with fish and seafood being recommended. This diet is usually prescribed by doctors to patients who suffer from chronic illnesses like high blood pressure and heart disease.

This eating plan is practiced in countries like Southern Italy, Crete, and Greece (NIH, 2021). People who live in these regions have been seen to have a higher life expectancy regardless of having limited healthcare access. Their type of food, together with regular exercise, have been credited with this long life expectancy. The pyramid shape does not give the specific proportions of the amount of food or nutrients that you must include per serving, it simply states that you need to eat more of this than that. For instance, it promotes eating more fruits and vegetables, as well as reducing dairy and animal protein intake. Every individual has to decide on the portion of the recommended foods to eat.

There are certain elements that make this diet unique. There is an emphasis on eating healthy fats with olive oil being used as the primary added oil and eliminating things like margarine and butter. In addition to eating olive oil, other foods that contain healthy fats high in Omega-3, such as walnuts, avocados, and oily fish, like sardines and salmon, can be included.

It is advised to include fish in your diet at least twice a week, then choose less of other animal protein like poultry, eggs, and dairy products like cheese and yogurt. Red meat can only be limited to a few times a month due to its effect of causing inflammation. Water is also used as the main beverage, however, wine is also allowed to drink during meals, with men taking two glasses per day, and women one glass per day. This meal must be accompanied by routine exercises through any enjoyable physical activity of your choice.

Advantages of Eating a Mediterranean Diet

In every diet, there are benefits which make people decide to follow it. The Mediterranean eating plan is not an exception, it is packed with its own advantages. Below are some of the benefits of eating a Mediterranean diet with various research evidence:

Overall Nutrition

One advantage of eating a Mediterranean diet is that it does not totally exclude any food group as it promotes the use of various nutrient-dense foods which means you can still enjoy flavors of different types of foods and at the same time get the required nutrients. The 2020-2025 Food Guidelines for Americans recommends the inclusion of healthy and nutritious food groups for individuals who are following the Mediterranean food plan and those who are considering the U.S. Style Dietary Pattern (Carol, 2019).

It is suggested that eating the required amounts of whole grain cereals, seafood, and dairy products, as well as drinking fortified soy beverages will make you gain enough vitamin D and calcium, which are all part of the Mediterranean diet.

Good Heart Health

A research study was conducted by scientists, checking the connection between the Mediterranean diet and heart health in controlled trials (Carol, 2019). They found that there was enough evidence to back up the fact that the Mediterranean diet is good for a healthy heart. Following this diet can result in reduced risk of heart attack, coronary heart disease, and mortality in general. The American Heart Association (AHA) promotes a food consumption style that reduces obesity, high cholesterol, diabetes, and high blood pressure (Carol, 2019).

Diabetes Control and Prevention

Those suffering from type 2 diabetes can significantly benefit from the Mediterranean diet by achieving better blood sugar control. About 56 trials were conducted on 4937 patients with type 2 diabetes between the years 1978 and 2016. The results indicated that the Mediterranean diet, in comparison to other controlled diets, is capable of lowering hemoglobin A1c levels (Carol, 2019).

This hemoglobin A1c shows the individual's blood sugar control for the past 3 months. Managing any blood sugar reduction is helpful no matter how small the margin is.

Hemoglobin A1c reflects the body's blood sugar control over the previous three months. Though a 0.32% reduction sounds small, any reduction may be helpful for people with diabetes who are trying to manage blood sugar levels. A study published in 2014 indicated that sticking to a Mediterranean diet can decrease the likelihood of being diagnosed with type 2 diabetes, with a lower carbohydrate intake of less than 50% per serving (Carol, 2019).

Improved Brain Health

One other benefit of the Mediterranean diet is better mental health and can lead to the reduction of clinical depression. It's a diet that emphasizes social relationships which is crucial for better mental health, especially in adult individuals. Keeping connections and maintaining social interactions can make you stay away from a feeling of loneliness, which is required for positive thinking and overall health.

Reduced Weight Maintenance

It may sound weird to tell someone that adding olive oil to your meals and eating nuts can help you reduce or maintain body weight. But, including this in your diet, in combination with foods rich in dietary fiber like fruits and vegetables can in actual fact help you stay full for a longer time. You won't crave more food, which will, in turn, lead to reduced weight. Sticking to this low-carbohydrate Mediterranean diet can restrict any weight gain, and for sure keep you out of the doctor's office as well.

Reduces Inflammation

When your finger is accidentally cut, it turns red and inflamed. If you hurt your knee, it also becomes swollen, red, and inflamed. So, if we talk of inflammation inside the body, what does it do to us? If you have little inflammation in your body, this can help facilitate your healing process. However, when inflammation becomes chronic, it can cause certain diseases in your body. Too much inflammation inside your body can cause damage to your brain, heart, and other important organs. Inflammation is the major culprit in causing diseases like cancer, depression, and Alzheimer's disease.

The same way we see some inflammation when we get hurt from outside the body is what happens even from within. Nevertheless, the truth of the matter is that what we put in our stomachs will determine the amount of inflammation that we get. Red meat and food that contain a lot of animal fat can lead to higher inflammation, as compared to eating seafood and food with healthy fats like avocado and nuts, which reduces the amount of inflammation.

Cancer Prevention

Cancer is not caused by a single factor, it's actually a combination of genetic, as well as environmental, factors. The food that we consume can also play a big role in causing this complex disease. Following the Mediterranean diet can help reduce the risk of cancer including liver cancer, colorectal cancer, gastric cancer, prostate cancer, and cancer of the neck.

Best for Our Environment

Relying on a plant-based diet and grains rather than eating beef and other red meats is good for the planet and its life. People are encouraged to consume a diet that is healthy for both humans and the planet. The organization promotes good patterns like the Mediterranean that are healthy and food for the planet. This type of diet conserves land, saves water, and avoids the use of fertilizers.

Disadvantages of Using a Mediterranean Diet

Other people can see some setbacks in this Mediterranean diet. Let's have a look at some of these disadvantages:

Some of the Food Can Be Costly

The Mediterranean diet does not include high-cost branded foods or even special supplements that may turn out to be expensive for you to buy. However, other consumers complain about the cost of certain items, including olive oil, nuts, seeds, and fish. If you scrutinize the price of seafood, it looks more expensive than other protein foods. But what you have to remember is that there are various ways to shop on a budget, inclusive of seafood.

For you to be able to save money, try and do your shopping sales from the grocery store. Let's take, for instance, a meal that requires a particular type of fish like locally caught cod and sea bass that can be found at a special price. Don't skip frozen seafood as it is cheaper than fresh seafood. After being thawed, it can cook very nicely. You may also opt to go for canned fish, which is less expensive as well.

More Guidance Is Required

For individuals with certain conditions like type 1 diabetes, additional guidance to the actual proportions or quantities of each food group may be required. Since the Mediterranean diet includes fruits and vegetables, if the amounts of carbohydrates consumed by these people are not monitored, there might be a spike in their sugar levels. Or, their sugar levels can drop abnormally low, which can cause problems for these patients.

It is vital for individuals with sugar diabetes to eat controlled amounts of carbohydrates throughout the day in order for them to stay away from trouble, especially those who use insulin or take oral medication. However, this diet can be very helpful to these patients, they simply have to find a dietician who can help to plan their Mediterranean diet accordingly.

Dealing With the Diet Restrictions May Be Challenging

Following the Mediterranean diet requires you to significantly reduce the consumption of red meat and added sugars, which some people might find quite challenging. Individuals on a Mediterranean diet are only allowed to eat these foods as a treat, a few times per month. This is contrary to those who are used to the standard American diet and consume added sugar all the time, which is found in processed foods.

But, you need to remember that having a diet with reduced sugars is of more benefit, so don't be scared to continue with the diet despite its reduced sugar restriction. It may sound better and easier to turn to a Western diet, which contains high amounts of added sugar, but this might have unpleasant consequences for you.

For the people who may find it difficult to eat red meat less frequently, they may opt for lean and unprocessed red meat, but in reduced quantities. Such portions of red meat may include brisket, flank, or top round.

Unsettled About the Amount of Alcohol Involved

The amount of alcohol consumption in this diet can be worrisome for certain individuals, especially the drinking of wine. Some people can still doubt if the consumption of this alcohol is really of any benefit. However, some experts believe it can be beneficial.

If alcohol is consumed as part of a well-balanced meal, it can be helpful. You simply need to also include regular movements as well as maintaining connections. The Mediterranean and other similar diets can teach us how to consume and enjoy alcohol in a healthy manner. This can help with cardiometabolic health and maintain positive social connections.

Chapter 2 has taken you through the Mediterranean diet. You now know what it means to follow this diet. In the next chapter, you will read about the Keto diet and have an understanding of what a keto diet is.

Chapter 3:

The Keto Diet

Keto is not a program that just fits everyone; it's about getting specifically what works for your particular body and lifestyle. —Amy Berger

In the previous chapter, you have read about the Mediterranean diet, its pros and cons, and the types of benefits that are included in it. This chapter is going to take you through the keto diet, its definition, and the types of food that this diet focuses on. I will also explain in detail what you benefit from this kind of diet, and what might be the disadvantages of following it.

The keto diet is one popular diet in the United States, but the question that is always asked is, is it safe? This is a diet that has a lot of celebrity endorsements and a bit more controversy. It is therefore difficult to rank it amongst other diets, as it lacks other vital nutrients.

Definition of the Keto Diet

A keto diet, also known as the ketogenic diet, refers to a high-fat, low-carb diet in which almost 90% of your calories come from the fat (Juma, 2023). The decreased carb intake only allows you to eat less than 50 grams of carbohydrates per meal (the average size of a banana can be 27 grams).

The aim of the keto diet is to push your body to use fat for energy, instead of using the usual glucose. When your body fails to get the required glucose, it goes into a ketosis state. In the beginning, this diet was prescribed to treat childhood epilepsy, however, it has recently become popular as a way to lose weight.

What types of food can you include in your keto diet? In this diet, you can think of all foods that contain a lot of fat: butter and cream, red meat, salmon, bacon, cheese, nuts, avocado, and olive oil. The diet may also include vegetables that contain fewer carbohydrates such as tomatoes, cucumbers, broccoli, or celery. However, the diet encourages an intake of less than 50 grams of carbohydrate consumption; therefore, you will have to avoid grains, fruits that contain too much glucose, starchy vegetables, baked foods, and anything with added sugars.

Who Can Go on the Keto Diet?

This diet is suitable for people who struggle with being overweight or trying to keep healthy blood sugar levels. This diet can help you kick-start the process and has proven to make people lose weight faster than someone on a traditional diet. For those who want to regulate their blood sugar levels, you need to first consult your healthcare provider to find out if this diet will be suitable for you.

Pros

Like any other diet, the keto diet has its own advantages that make its followers choose it and not the others. Let's find out what people like about the keto diet:

Reduced Appetite

It is more appetite or hunger that messes with our eagerness to lose weight. Feeling hungry when you are trying to lose weight may be the biggest obstacle when it comes to achieving your goals, making it the reason a lot of people give up and start to eat their normal, traditional diet again.

However, what you need to understand is that, when you reduce carbohydrate consumption from your meals, this means an appetite reduction. When you cut down on your carbohydrate consumption and replace them with healthy fats and proteins, you are bound to eat less. This is because protein and fats take longer to be digested in your stomach; therefore, you feel fuller for a longer amount of time.

Weight Loss Due to Less Carbs

Reducing the amount of carbohydrate intake can significantly reduce your weight during the initial stages. Individuals on a low-carb diet lose weight faster than those on a low-fat diet, besides the fact that a low-fat diet also restricts calories. This is true because a low-carb diet can help to get rid of excess fluids from your body, thereby reducing insulin levels and causing you to quickly lose weight during the initial stages of the diet. When comparing a low-carb diet with a low-fat diet, those restricting their carb intake lose much more weight and don't feel as hungry.

More Fat Is Lost From the Abdomen

The area where your body fat is stored greatly determines how it affects your health and the risk level of suffering from certain diseases. There are two basic types of this fat: the first one is subcutaneous, which is usually found under the skin, and visceral fat, the one that is found in the abdomen. Most overweight men have more visceral fat accumulated within their abdominal cavity.

The more dangerous type of fat is the visceral type because it accumulates around the human organs which may lead to metabolic dysfunction. Having excess visceral fat in your body can cause more inflammation as well as insulin resistance. Sticking to a low-carb diet can help you to lessen this unwanted and harmful abdominal fat. People on a low-carb diet lose more fat from their abdominal cavity. In the long run, this can prevent you from having heart disease or suffering from type 2 sugar diabetes.

Reduced Triglycerides

When we talk of triglycerides, we refer to fat molecules that are found circulating in your bloodstream. These triglycerides can become a big risk to the heart after fasting, even after fasting overnight, as their levels are high. Individuals who practice a sedentary lifestyle are also at high risk, the triglycerides levels are elevated by high carbohydrate consumption. When people reduce the amount of carbohydrate intake, especially simple sugar fructose, there will be a significant reduction in the levels of blood triglycerides.

Surprisingly, low-fat diets can also cause the level of triglycerides to rise because food without or with less fat can make you feel hungry fast, and you get to eat more carbohydrates to kill hunger. In the case of the keto diet, consuming less carbohydrates and more fat helps you to stay full for a long time, hence a lower level of triglycerides.

Higher Amounts of Good HDL Cholesterol

Good cholesterol, also known as High-density lipoprotein (HDL) can help you to reduce the risk of heart disease. If you have higher levels of HDL and less Low-density Lipoprotein (LDL), you are less likely to suffer from heart disease. The fastest way to increase your good HDL amounts is to consume more fat and reduce carbohydrate consumption. Funny enough, HDL levels tend to increase significantly for individuals on a low-carb diet, when they increase slightly or rather decrease for people on low-fat diets.

Lower Blood Sugar Levels

Individuals struggling with sugar diabetes and insulin resistance can also benefit from this low-carb ketogenic diet. When diabetic people cut their carbohydrate consumption, they drastically reduce both their insulin levels and blood sugar. Those diabetic individuals who are taking blood sugar medication, you need to talk to your healthcare provider first before you can implement any changes to the amount of carbohydrates that you eat. You may need to have your dosage adjusted to avoid hypoglycemia.

Can Reduce Blood Pressure

When you suffer from high blood pressure, this can also put you at a high risk of developing other diseases like renal failure, stroke, and heart disease. Going on a low-carb diet can help you prevent these diseases and hence increase your life expectancy.

Fight Against Metabolic Syndrome

Suffering from metabolic syndrome can also make you susceptible to heart disease, as well as diabetes. Metabolic symptoms can be diagnosed if you show symptoms of high blood pressure, abdominal obesity, elevated levels of triglycerides, and low levels of good HDL cholesterol. But, when you begin a low-carb diet, you can reduce the risk of suffering from all these illnesses.

Reduced Levels of Bad LDL Cholesterol

If you have higher levels of bad LDL, you are at a risk of suffering a heart attack. Whether you are at risk of heart attack or not depends on the size of their particles; with smaller particles putting you at a higher risk of heart attack and the bigger particles being linked to reduced risk. When you eat a low-carb diet, that can increase the size of bad LDL particles while, at the same time, reducing the amount of LDL particles in your bloodstream. This can in turn help you improve your heart health.

Therapy for Mental Disorders

Glucose is required by some parts of the brain to function well, as these parts can only burn this type of sugar. If you don't get enough glucose in your body, your liver can end up producing glucose from proteins to ensure that your brain parts are being the amount of glucose required. However, the larger part of the brain can burn ketones, which are produced when the body is starved or the carbohydrate consumption is very low. You can see the logic behind the keto diet.

Cons

There are negative effects that come with drastic changes in diet. If you don't follow the diet correctly or use it for too long, this diet can come with unwanted effects. Let's have a look at the disadvantages of taking a keto diet:

Dehydration

A keto diet can result in the loss of water before the person can even start to lose fat. Therefore, when starting to follow this diet, the first side effect that you will experience is dehydration.

You become dehydrated when your body loses too many fluids, which means you will be losing fluids at a faster rate than you take in. Signs and symptoms of dehydration include dry mouth or throat, passing dark-colored urine, tiredness, dizziness, and always feeling thirsty.

Gastrointestinal Problems

Another side effect of following a keto diet is gastrointestinal (GI) issues such as diarrhea, vomiting, constipation, and nausea. You can experience diarrhea more frequently due to high-fat content meals, which the body may struggle to absorb quickly.

Kidney Stones

The high-fat foods associated with the keto diet can also lead you to suffer from kidney stones, which are mineral-formed substances. People who have never shown any problems with their kidneys may start to form kidney stones as a side effect of the keto diet.

If someone is already suffering from kidney issues, following a keto diet might cause more damage to their kidneys. They can also suffer from metabolic acidosis, which is most likely the cause of the formation of kidney stones. This is because of the reduced citrate and pH levels, as well as high levels of calcium in the urine.

Poor Athletic Performance

Athletes who follow the ketogenic diet may rejoice in weight loss and enhanced sports activities. However, it was discovered that a keto diet can result in worse performance on high-intensity running tasks four days after starting the diet.

Causes Keto Flu

Certain individuals can start experiencing the keto flu after beginning this diet. When you have keto flu, you are more likely to have symptoms like finding it difficult to exert yourself during exercises, fatigue, dizziness, constipation, nausea, and vomiting.

To reduce the likelihood of developing the keto flu, it is advised to drink lots of water and increase your electrolyte intake. Another trick to avoid the flu is to slowly reduce your carbohydrate intake bit by bit, rather than a drastic reduction, thus easing your way into the diet and macro requirements.

May Lack Other Nutrients

Taking the keto diet can force you to limit the fruits and vegetables you eat in order to lower the amount of carbohydrate intake. This will result in your body receiving inadequate nutrients such as fiber calcium, potassium, iron, and magnesium. In addition to this, individuals on a keto diet can also fall short of other nutrients like vitamins A, B, C, E, and K, as well as thiamin and folate. These nutrients are crucial for the human body's development of bones, red blood cells, and gums.

Increased Body Weight

When you stop following the keto diet, you are bound to gain the weight back—and, possibly, more than you lost. The reason is that weight loss is difficult to sustain. A person is recommended to follow a diet for at least 3 weeks up to one year. It is always advised to see a dietician before you embark on a dieting journey so that you are guided through the process.

This chapter has taken you through the keto diet, the types of food that you can consume during the dieting period, and who is suitable for this lifestyle change. In Chapter 4, we will discuss the plant-based diet. I'm sure the name says it all, so let's continue reading.

Chapter 4:

The Plant-Based Diet

As we move on to learning about different types of diets, you may be starting to see your favorite diets. In Chapter 3, you learned about the ketogenic diet, why you should try it, and why it might not be suitable for you. This chapter will take us through the plant-based diet, the food that it focuses on eating, and which foods are not advised to consume when following it. We will also look at the reasons why this diet is good, as well as its side effects.

What Is a Plant-Based Diet?

When we talk of a plant-based diet, we refer to a diet that consists mainly of foods that come from plants. The diet includes a variety of dietary patterns with very little amounts of animal products but focuses on plant products like whole grains, fruits, vegetables, seeds, and nuts. The idea here is not to say you don't touch meat or animal products but to minimize them and focus more on plant-based foods.

Some people may think of a plant-based diet as a different way of eating, and others choose to use the words "plant-based" and "vegetarian" interchangeably. Does this mean one is totally removing animal foods from their diet or there is another explanation? To be more clear, here we are talking about a diet plan that focuses on consuming foods that come from plants, including foods that contain a lot of nutrients. However, the diet must contain a larger portion of the foods from plants.

If we say the plant-based diet consists of whole grains, fruits and vegetables and more, does that mean it's good to eat things like refined grains, sugars, and vegan fast foods? These may be plant-based, but they shouldn't be referred to as healthy. We are talking about a plant-based diet that focuses on healthy eating and balancing the diet, therefore, choosing to eat more of the good and healthy stuff and reduce the bad ones.

What Are the Various Kinds of Plant-Based Diets?

The main plant-based diets are:

- **The vegetarian diet:** There is no consumption of meat, poultry, or even seafood.

- **The vegan diet:** This type of plant-based diet eliminates the inclusion of animal products such as meat, dairy, seafood, poultry, and eggs.

- **Plant-based whole food diet:** This diet does not allow the consumption of any animal products and does not include plant-based foods that are highly processed.

"I am a newbie on the plant-based diet, I don't know where to start." Your concerns are understood, check below for all the tips that you require to get started:

- **One of the secrets of this diet is to eat lots of vegetables**: When you sit down to eat your lunch or dinner, half of your plate should be filled with vegetables. Deep-colored vegetables contain more nutrients, so make sure you include a variety of colorful vegetables in your meal.

- **You need to have a different mindset about meat**: Serve it in smaller quantities, as a garnish or in your salad—not as the centerpiece of your meal.

- **Make a good selection of healthy fats**: Get your fats from things like olive oil, nuts, seeds and avocados. Most of these items contain Omega-3 fatty acids, which are good for your health.

- **Try to make a vegetarian meal at least once or twice a week**: Make use of healthy foods like whole grains, beans, and vegetables.

- **Start your day by eating whole grains for breakfast**: For example, oatmeal, barley, or quinoa. Improve and make your breakfast enjoyable by adding fresh fruits, seeds, or nuts.

- **Add more dark green vegetables to your diet**: These vegetables include leafy vegetables like spinach, kale, Swiss chard, and many more. Use cooking methods that will preserve most of the nutrients like steaming, brazing, or grilling.

- **Build your** meal around a salad: Your salad bowl should have lots of salad greens, like romaine, cucumber, or res leafy greens.

- **Find a healthy fruit that you want after a meal**: Some of your best options include a slice of watermelon or an apple.

What Are the Benefits of a Plant-based Diet?

We have a lot of benefits for choosing a plant-based diet, which are all science-based. The following is a list of advantages of going on a plant-based diet:

Excellent Weight Management

Following a plant-based diet makes you lose weight, as well as have a leaner and more manageable body. It becomes easier for you to engage in any type of sporting activity than someone who is not on a diet. Because the diet is filled with more dietary fiber, you can eat more without having to significantly increase your amount of calorie intake.

Prevent Diseases

Stay away from the doctor by eating a plant-based diet. Eating whole foods and plant-based foods can prevent you from having certain diseases and in other instances can reverse some chronic illnesses. This diet has a history of preventing heart diseases and diabetes as well as reduced rates of arthritis and kidney problems.

When it comes to a healthy heart, a plant-based diet plays a big role in proper cardiovascular functioning. Since this diet is rich in unprocessed plant-based foods, it was seen as being able to reduce cardiovascular diseases as compared to other diets that include meat and dairy products. Staying away from highly processed foods and meat prevents blood cholesterol from rising, which may cause fatty, wax-like plaque to accumulate and block the free movement of blood in the arteries.

The higher amounts of salt contained in processed foods can also cause health problems such as blood pressure and damage to the lining of the arteries. Removing these unhealthy foods and replacing them with whole plant-based foods will be a good move since they reduce blood pressure and heart disease.

This diet was found to work better for those with diabetes and people's overall well-being than other foods that are recommended by various diabetes associations. The plant-based diet excludes the consumption of saturated fats, which have been known to cause insulin resistance. When this diet prevents you from becoming obese, it also helps you avoid diabetes since type 2 diabetes thrives more in people suffering from obesity.

Good for the Planet

The consumption of a plant-based diet has more benefits besides what it can do for the human body; it also helps the environment. When we look at animal-based foods, we first have to raise poultry and livestock, occupying land resources. If we eliminate this middleman part, by not first feeding these animals in order to eat them, but rather to eat the plant-based foods directly, we are doing our part for the planet.

Saves Money

Besides whole plant-based foods being healthy, they are cheaper than most items in your grocery basket. According to the Journal of Hunger and Environmental Nutrition, eating a whole plant-based diet can save you around $750 per year (Forks Over Knives, 2017). For the people who like backyard farming, they can easily grow some of the plants for themselves so that they don't have to buy these foods.

Disadvantages of Going on a Plant-based Diet

Despite having so many advantages of eating a whole plant-based diet, there are also some disadvantages of following this diet. Let's check them out:

Possibility of Not Eating Enough Protein

It may be difficult for you to make a well-balanced whole plant based meal, particularly if you are on a strict vegetarian or vegan diet. It may be challenging to know what nutrients are making up your meal unless you carefully plan them out, maybe with the help of a dietician. If you fail to do so, you may not be able to meet your daily protein requirements.

For you to obtain the required amount of protein in your meal, you must include more foods like beans, seeds, legumes, nuts, and whole grains. If you usually eat away from home, it might be a challenge to ensure you are eating protein-rich foods. You might have to prepare a packed lunch to make sure that wherever you eat throughout the day, you stick to your diet and won't be tempted to eat what's not on your diet list. You may also have to buy and eat food from restaurants that specialize in whole plant-based and nutrient-balanced meals.

Labels of Plant-Based May Fool You

The foods that we buy from the shops can confuse and fool customers into thinking that they are healthy when they're actually not. Suppliers and manufacturers of foods may mislead customers simply because they want to improve their sales. The label has to clearly indicate "p lant-*based*" to show that it really is the product you want to buy.

The other thing that you need to know is that when food is labeled "*plant-based*," it doesn't mean it's regulated and suppliers don't have to meet any criteria to be able to print such a label. Also, take note that any supplier who puts such a label on their products will do it out of its own nutritional profile. To make sure you aren't being fooled by the misleading labels, read over the ingredient list and nutritional fact panels to find out how healthy the product you are buying really is.

You Might Need to Supplement Some Nutrients

You could be required to supplement other important nutrients that you might be lacking in your diet. Although you might be eating a well-balanced whole plant-based diet, it's possible to fall short when it comes to receiving other essential nutrients. The reason is that we have certain nutrients that are packed in animal products and very minimal in plant foods. For instance, vitamin B12 can be found in abundance in animal products but scarce in plant foods, often only being obtained from fortified soy milk or yeast.

We also have other nutrients that are difficult to get from a plant-based diet like vitamin D. This vitamin can be found in fatty fish and fortified dairy products, which are restricted on a vegan diet. We can also obtain vitamin A from mushrooms, fortified plant-based juices, and cereals, as well as basking in the sunshine. The fact that there are only a few plant-based foods that contain vitamin D makes it vital for people on a plant-based diet to look for vitamin D supplements.

Take care of your iron intake as well. Plant-based foods contain iron in abundance, but the type of iron present in these foods is not absorbed by your body the same way that animal fat does. The iron that is present in animal products, and not in plant-based food items, is referred to as non-heme. To improve the absorption of plant-based iron by your body, you need to combine them with diet-approved foods that are high in vitamin C. For example, you could pair your broccoli with tofu or peppers with lentils.

Requires a Lot of Planning

To successfully meet the nutrient requirements of a plant-based diet, you need enough time to plan out your meals and snacks. This means you have to spare a lot of time which a lot of people might find difficult.

Plant–Based Foods Are Perishable

Vegetables and fruits can easily go bad, so you need to buy them for short periods since you can't keep them ripe for a long time. Visiting the store more frequently can also be tiring and time-consuming.

Vegetarian and Vegan Diets Restrict Meat Consumption

Those who are on vegan or vegetarian diets are not allowed to consume animal products, which some individuals may find difficult to stick to.

Hooray! You now know if you could consider going for a whole plant-based diet or the other diets that we have discussed in the previous chapters. In the next chapter, you are going to learn about the paleo diet, its definition, and the types of foods that it focuses on.

Chapter 5:

The Paleolithic Diet

Consuming a Paleolithic diet is not about historical re-enactment; it is about mimicking the effect of such a diet on the metabolism of foods available at the supermarket. There was no consumed diet eaten throughout the whole Paleolithic period, nor was there ever a single diet taken by contemporary hunter-gatherers. Hunter-gatherer diets can vary substantially depending on the geography, season, and culture. Besides that, the commonalities among the hunter-gatherer diets give useful parameters for a healthy modern diet. —John Durant

Chapter 4 has taken you through all the processes that you need to follow in order to successfully benefit from a whole plant-based diet. You now know where to start and where to end when going for a plant-based diet. In this chapter, we are going to discuss the Paleo diet, its definition, and what is consumed by its followers. We shall also discuss the merits and demerits of going on the Paleo diet.

The Paleo diet is the original diet that was eaten by our ancestors, the hunter-gatherers from the time humans appeared on this planet. When we eat the Paleo diet, we eat the diet that was originally programmed in our DNA.

Most of the foods that were eaten a long time ago no longer exist in this day, so the Paleo diet that exists tries to mimic the "old day" diet. Despite the Paleo diet having been founded by Dr. Loren Cordain, he was quite clear about emphasizing that he is not the original creator of this diet—but, rather, it was our ancestors. Cordain and his colleagues only discovered the science behind this diet decades ago (The Paleo Diet, 2020).

When comparing the Paleo diet and a traditional Western diet, the Western diet has only been implemented decades ago. This diet brought up processed foods, refined sugars, and vegetable oils. Even today, our bodies have not yet adjusted to modern diets; but if we eat the Paleo diet, you would see that this is the diet that the human body is adapted to thrive on. With the Paleo diet, you eat nutrient-dense foods like fruits and vegetables, seafood, and lean meats. This diet does not promote the consumption of unhealthy foods such as processed foods, dairy products, refined sugars, and oils, which usually cause inflammation in humans.

We have different types of fad diets that have surfaced and disappeared while the Paleo diet is here to stay. It is one of the science-based diets, which medical professionals have approved since it is a reality-based diet. Americans like to rely on eating so much processed foods, which is why the Paleolithic diet is becoming a favorite to many as it represents the diet that our ancestors used to eat. They weren't eating cookies, so should we? The choice of a diet that our ancestors used to eat makes us enjoy a manageable body weight and healthy life.

Definition of a Paleo Diet

The Paleo diet mimics our ancestral diet, which included whole unprocessed foods like seeds, nuts, vegetables, fruits, and lean meat. It might be difficult to pinpoint the exact type of food that our ancestors used to eat around the globe, but what is known is that the diet consisted of whole foods. The Paleo diet helps to reduce body weight and the risk of having certain illnesses like obesity. Because of this kind of diet, coupled with a lot of physical activities, our ancestral hunter-gatherers avoided suffering from lifestyle illnesses like diabetes and heart disease.

Who, then, is suitable for the Paleo diet? If this is the food that our ancestors hunted and gathered for consumption, it means that everyone can eat it. Those who want to lose weight and are ready to make their meals from scratch would be perfect for this diet as it consists of grass-fed meat, wild-caught seafood, fresh produce, and eggs. However, foods from grains are not recommended, therefore, making it a gluten-free diet.

Who Can Benefit From Being on a Paleo Diet?

Individuals who struggle to follow diets that require them to count calories can turn to the Paleolithic diet. The diet is not very easy to follow though, as there are certain foods that are restricted making it difficult for some people who enjoy eating the restricted items. The meals also require diligent preparation and cooking.

The Paleo diet was founded as a way to reduce the likelihood of type 2 diabetes as well as heart-related illnesses, so patients who are borderline or at risk can also go for this diet.

Benefits of The Paleo Diet

It is widely believed that the Paleo diet has therapeutic benefits, both emotionally and physically when it comes to metabolic diseases, mental health, and autoimmune problems. Most chronic diseases respond favorably to the Paleo diet since it has anti-inflammatory effects. Let's check out the principles and benefits of this diet.

It's Accepted by Our DNA

Cutting down on processed foods and added sugars and focusing on whole foods, which are the foods that our bodies are ready to eat and digest without problems.

Enhance Nutrient Density

The Paleolithic diet promotes the consumption of nutrient-dense foods. For example, blueberries, salmon, and green leafy vegetables. This is not what we get when eating the Western diet, which involves eating fatty meats, dairy products, refined sugars, and processed foods. Following the Paleo diet means you have to eliminate all these unhealthy foods and replace them with foods promoted by the Paleo diet, which are packed with vitamins, phytochemicals, and minerals.

Does Not Focus on Quantities, Only on Healthy Foods

Those who follow the Paleo diet don't need to bother themselves with the ratio of food nutrients that make up their meal. This is in line with the way our ancestors used to eat; it didn't matter how much protein, in comparison with carbohydrates or other nutrients, could make a meal. The same goes for the Paleo diet; it only focuses on eating healthy foods, not how much of each nutrient. What we simply know is that the more healthy natural foods you consume, the more protein and fewer carbohydrates you get, which the Western diet does not do.

No Cravings Are Experienced

Consuming the foods recommended for the Paleolithic diet is one way to get rid of regular cravings. The fact that your body gets the kind of food it likes significantly reduces the hunger signals. This is achieved by controlling and stabilizing insulin levels while, at the same time, improving your glycemic control, which is a great benefit for diabetic patients.

Consuming more simple sugars also increases the calorie intake and spikes hunger signals, making it a rotational cycle. Those who follow the Paleolithic diet eat fewer calories while getting the nutrients that the body requires. You will, therefore, remain energetic, eliminate cravings, and have a controlled body weight.

Reduce Energy Fluctuations

The Paleo diet promotes the consumption of foods that have a lower glycemic load. By glycemic load, we mean the rate at which a meal affects the blood and insulin levels. The good thing about the Paleolithic diet is that it contains less glycemic load.

Promotes the Consumption of Natural Foods

The nature of the Paleo diet will ensure that you consume more natural foods, in their natural form, and less processed ones. This is because the diet includes fruits, vegetables, seeds, nuts, and fish. Some people say the Paleo diet focuses on the consumption of meat, which is not factual; however, this diet is not a vegetarian diet despite the fact that it is heavily dependent on plant-based foods.

Maintains Important Nutrient Ratios

Our bodies require certain nutrients to be balanced, and it is the Paleo diet that can provide the balance that is well accepted by our bodies. A good example is the sodium-potassium ratio the Paleolithic diet provides, which is generally the amount required by our bodies. This is, however, contrary to the Western diet which has a sodium-potassium ratio that sits at 10:1. Our bodies actually require a ratio of 1:2. The Paleolithic diet does not promote added salts or any sea salt, which makes it more favorable.

The consumption of higher sodium in relation to potassium can cause higher acid levels in the body, which negatively impacts our health. It is believed that higher levels of sodium in one's diet can cause a condition known as osteoporosis. The Paleo diet also maintains a good ratio of magnesium-calcium, which also can negatively affect our health if consumed in the wrong ratios.

Provides the Correct Ratios of Fatty Acids

There was an incorrect belief that the consumption of any type of fat has an adverse effect on the human body. However, this was due to insufficient research or misleading information. The fact of the matter is, it is the type of fat that you consume that matters, along with the ratio of omega-6 to omega-3 fatty acids. The foods like fish, nuts, fruits, and vegetables included in the Paleo diet automatically supply the required ratio.

Helps to Improve the Acid-Base Balance

The consumption of lots of vegetables in the Paleo diet can increase potassium and help reduce the risk of osteoporosis. The Western diet is known for being acidic, which causes inflammation; and this inflammation can also cause osteoporosis.

Cut Off Anti-Nutrient

Consumption of grains that contain anti-nutrients, like wheat, can cause problems for human health. These anti-nutrients include saponins and lectins and they can evade one's intestinal defense, causing you to feel ill if the grains are consumed raw.

When you cook your grains, this will reduce the amount of anti-nutrients and this is not good again. It is believed that the remaining small amounts of anti-nutrients can still cause health problems. They cause high inflammation, which can lead to inflammatory diseases such as cancer. The Paleo diet, however, eliminates grain foods that contain anti-nutrients.

Enjoy Your Freedom

The types of food you eat on a Paleolithic diet will fill you with happiness. This is because natural foods will leave you feeling energetic and stabilize you physically, as well as emotionally. This new lifestyle can reward you on a daily basis as you become more confident.

Demerits of the Paleolithic Diet

A Paleolithic diet has a lot of health benefits for those who are on this diet; however, there may be some setbacks that you can also find in this diet. There's a fear that individuals who are following the Paleolithic diet might run short of certain nutrients, such as vitamins, fiber, and other key nutrients. Failure to consume food like whole grains, legumes, and dairy products may cause deficiencies in nutrients such as vitamin B, vitamin D, and calcium. When you continue lacking these nutrients, this can put you at risk of suffering from osteoporosis.

Buying some of the foods that are recommended in the Paleo diet seems to be more expensive than when you buy without any restrictions. Foods like fresh fish and meat can be more expensive than processed foods, such as canned and frozen foods. Meals can be difficult to plan when you don't have some of the foods that are left out of the Paleo diet and have to depend on fresh foods only.

Watch out for the low-carb flu, an illness also referred to as *the* "keto flu," which is related to consuming an inadequate amount of carbohydrates. Certain individuals can start experiencing symptoms such as fatigue, nausea, and headaches when their bodies are trying to adjust to the Paleolithic diet.

This diet might not be for everyone due to certain restrictions, just like the total elimination of some food groups may not be the best thing for other people. The fact that you just eat without measuring how much of each food group you are consuming can lead to the unnecessary consumption of huge amounts of some foods, yet other food groups will be lacking. However, you are advised to consult your healthcare provider before embarking on a journey of following this diet.

Today, people are no longer genetically identical to our Stone Age ancestors during the Paleolithic period. Most of the things have changed and we now have to adapt to the current environment and the types of food that are currently available. Most of the plants and animals that existed during the Paleolithic period have changed and we also have to consume what is currently available for us. Therefore, this Paleolithic diet does not have enough evidence as to how much food was being consumed during that period.

Now that we are done with Chapter 5, you have a full understanding of what a Paleolithic diet is. It's up to you to decide if you want to make it one of your favorites or not. In the next chapter, you're going to read about the DASH diet, its definition, and the individuals suitable for it.

Chapter 6:

The DASH Diet

One good, but difficult, way to prevent wrinkles is to stop smoking. Every puff you get contains a lot of free radicals. Nicotine suffocates the skin, causing it to deteriorate. Cigarettes have thousands of toxins that damage elastin and collagen, the proteins that improve your skin and make it look taut and wrinkle-free. The action of smoking—and its puckering and taking out the smoke—also makes ugly wrinkles, those that come from repetitive motion. Stay away from smoking to avoid further damage, and give the chance to the DASH diet's good nutrition to start improving your skin. —Marla Heller

In chapter 5, we have discussed the Paleolithic diet, why you should eat it, and why you shouldn't. We have also talked about the advantages that make this diet favorable and the possible setbacks that might make other people stay away from it. In this chapter, we are going to cover the DASH diet, its definitions, and the kind of people who are recommended to try it. We will also look at the types of foods that this diet focuses on, as well as the ones that are not recommended.

What Are the Advantages and Disadvantages of the Dash Diet?

The DASH diet is there to guide you in eating nutritious foods. Besides being a traditional "low-salt" diet, this diet emphasizes foods that lower blood pressure, such as foods that contain higher amounts of magnesium, fiber, potassium, and calcium. On top of recommending healthy eating, the DASH diet also promotes exercise and engaging in physical activities for at least 30 minutes a day, primarily on days that cover the bigger part of the week. You can aim your exercises at reaching 2 hours and 30 minutes per week of activities at an average intensity (NIH, 2021). You need to make sure you do cardiovascular exercises to get your heart pumping. If you wish to avoid weight gain, try and increase your exercise time to at least 60 minutes a day.

To successfully follow the DASH diet to lose weight, you must eat fruits and vegetables that don't contain starch. Also, eat average portions of foods like:

- Dairy products that contain less fat or those that are actually fat-free

- Fresh fish

- Whole-grain foods

- Beans, legumes, soy foods, lean meat, eggs, and poultry

- Seeds and nuts

- Fats that help with heart health, like avocados and olive oil

You should also try to eat less of:

- Foods that contain high saturated fats, such as fatty meals, full-fat dairy products, and tropical oils

- Sugar-added beverages and sweets

- Consuming large amounts of alcohol

Your dietician or healthcare provider can help you calculate the amount of calories that you can consume per day. The amount of your calorie intake per day will highly depend on how active you are, your gender, your previous medical conditions, and whether you want to maintain the weight that you have or lose it. The DASH diet promotes eating smaller portions and swapping other healthy foods to encourage weight loss.

Definition of a DASH Diet

DASH means Dietary Approaches to Stop Hypertension. A DASH diet refers to a healthy eating plan that was developed to prevent high blood pressure or treat it for those who already have it. This diet can also be used to lower cholesterol levels, which is associated with heart disease (NIH, 2021). The DASH diet is focused on the consumption of whole foods, which include whole grains, fish, poultry, beans, nuts, and low-fat dairy products. This diet is considered to be heart-friendly since it consists of low amounts of saturated and trans fats, as well as reduced refined sugar. However, it promotes the intake of calcium, magnesium, fiber, and antioxidants, all of which help with the health function of the heart. Going on this diet could significantly lower blood pressure for those who are struggling to do so using alternative methods.

Being able to manage your LDL cholesterol levels and reduce high blood pressure means also reduced risk of heart disease and stroke. The aim of this diet is not to lose weight but to reduce blood pressure. However, the moment you go on this diet, you will automatically lose weight, lower cholesterol levels, and prevent diabetes.

Those who enjoy eating a lot of salt will be forced to significantly reduce it if they want to go on the DASH diet. The standard diet restricts salt intake to 2,300 mg a day, the same amount that is recommended in the Dietary Guidelines for Americans.

When you are starting the DASH diet, you are recommended to consume a specific number of servings per day from different food groups. Knowing the number of servings you need per day will depend on the specific quantity of calories that you are recommended to consume.

It is advisable to make gradual changes, starting with lower amounts of sodium, during the initial stages. Then, you can adjust and further reduce the amount as you get used to eating meals with less salt. You could also start by limiting yourself to 2,300 mg of sodium in one day, which measures about 1 teaspoon. If you see that your body is now used to this amount, you can further reduce the amount and make it 1,500 mg per day, which is about two-thirds of a teaspoon (NIH, 2021). This limit must include all the salt that you use in your food, including the salt that is already in the products that you buy, the ingredients that you cook with, and the meals that you add when eating at the table. Let's have a look at some of the tips for the DASH diet:

- Include fruits in your meals. You can use canned or dried fruits as they are easy to use

- Make sure you include vegetables for both your lunch and dinner

- Reduce the amount of butter, margarine, or salad dressing by almost half, and you may opt to use fat-free condiments or the ones with low-fat

- Replace full-fat dairy products with low-fat or skimmed milk

- Restrict the amount of your meat intake to six ounces

- Make beans part of your diet

- For snacks, you can eat unsalted popcorn without butter, unsalted nuts, and pretzels. Avoid eating chips and sweets for your snacks.

- Make sure you read food labels to know the amount of salt that the food contains

Benefits of a DASH Diet

The DASH diet was implemented during the 90s when they were trying to find natural therapy for high blood pressure (NIH, 2021). It was seen that the DASH diet could help to reduce high blood pressure, even without considering the weight loss part and decreased sodium intake. However, choosing to go for the more restricted diet for weight loss, which strictly limits sodium intake, can tremendously reduce high blood pressure. The following are some of the benefits of eating a DASH diet:

Easy Access

The DASH diet recommends people eat foods that are easy to access and are found in most food stores. All the foods on the list are not hard-to-get ingredients, foods, subscriptions, or supplements for those on the program. For this diet, you can find everything you want to know about it online, free of charge, which may not be the same as other diet plans. Another source of information for the DASH diet is the National Institute of Health, where you can get a full guide to suggested servings, sodium intake, calorie guides, meal plans, and cooking recipes.

You can also get various cooking books and phone apps that support this diet. Since it is a well-known diet with information available everywhere, the chances are high that your healthcare provider could be familiar with it. This means if you need guidance or have any questions about how to follow the diet, they will have the information at their fingertips.

It's a Flexible Diet

This diet is meant for both men and women with different calorie requirements, depending on their level of activity. Individuals who are on special diets can easily go for the DASH diet. Let's take, for example, people who are on a vegan or vegetarian diet. They would be able to easily follow the program since it includes foods like fruits, vegetables, and grains.

For gluten-free dieters, they have an option to choose to consume safe grains like quinoa and buckwheat. The DASH diet can also be taken by people who eat a halal diet, as they can simply choose the foods that conform to their standards while, at the same time, following the DASH diet plan.

A Well-Balanced Diet

If you look at the DASH diet, it doesn't restrict a whole food group like what other diets do, such as low-diet and low-carb diets. It's one diet that maintains a balance of nutrients and stays within the limits provided by the United States Department of Agriculture (USDA). For instance, the DASH diet recommends the consumption of about 55% carbohydrate calories, while the USDA recommends eating between 45% and 65% of carbohydrate calories (NIH, 2021). This finds the DASH diet to be within the recommended limit.

On the other hand, the USDA also recommends that between 20% and 35% of the calories that you consume must come from fat, and approximately 10% of that calories must be saturated fat. When following the DASH diet, you are not permitted to have more than 27% of your calorie consumption coming from fat, while about 6% of the calories would be saturated (NIH, 2021). While following the program, you're supposed to also meet the other nutrient requirements like calcium, fiber, and protein.

Reduced Cholesterol Levels

One benefit of the DASH diet is its ability to improve the markers of bad cholesterol as well as triglycerides. A high unsaturated fats DASH diet, which substitutes almost 10% of the carbohydrates with fat, was seen to effectively lower LDL cholesterol, high blood, or triglycerides the same way as the original diet, yet without lowering the HDL cholesterol (NIH, 2021).

Can Reduce the Risk of Heart Disease

The fact that the DASH diet significantly reduces high blood pressure levels, we all understand that the lower blood pressure, the lower the risk of cardiovascular diseases. The diet can lower the risk of stroke by 19% and heart failure by 29% (NIH, 2021).

Weight Reduction

When it comes to losing weight, people who are overweight and obese are welcome to try the DASH diet. It's good for weight control and it was seen to be more helpful than the calorie-restricted standard American diet.

Help to Reduce Type 2 Diabetes

The DASH diet is also beneficial for individuals with type 2 diabetes since it helps to lower sugar levels. This diet can improve insulin sensitivity for people who want to change their lifestyle and couple this diet with regular exercises and weight loss.

Improved Metabolic Syndrome

When you have metabolic syndrome, you tend to suffer from the following issues: abdominal obesity, high blood pressure, high triglycerides, and low HDL cholesterol. The DASH diet can help you to improve these biomarkers and result in the prevention and management of metabolic syndrome.

Reduced Risk of Cancer

The DASH diet promotes the consumption of foods that are high in vitamins, antioxidants, mineral elements, and fiber, which gives it the power to fight cancer. Antioxidants are chemicals that help to stop the formation of cancer by neutralizing free radicals that damage the cells. These antioxidants can also be referred to as "free radical scavengers."

Your body is capable of creating its own antioxidants that can be used to neutralize free radicals. However, the body depends largely on external sources of antioxidants, particularly the diet, to get the antioxidants required to fight the free radicals. Other sources of antioxidants include vitamins A, C, and D, beta-carotene, and lycopene.

Let's check out what these cancer-causing free radicals really are. Free radicals refer to highly reactive chemicals which are capable of damaging our cells. These are formed when a molecule or an atom, at some point, either loses or gains an electron (a tiny negatively charged particle). Free radicals are naturally created inside the body and are used in several normal processes in the cells. But, if you have huge amounts of free radicals, they can damage your cells, including cell membranes and the DNA. This cell damage can then lead to the formation of cancer, particularly damage to the DNA.

Can Reduce the Risk of Gout

A DASH diet's ability to lower serum uric acid amounts can help to lower the risk of gout. Gout is known to be a metabolic disease, which usually occurs in conjunction with cardiovascular diseases and high blood pressure; therefore, the diet can also help to heal all these illnesses.

Can Help With Kidney Health

Consuming less processed foods and red meat, coupled with a higher intake of healthy foods like legumes, nuts, and reduced-fat dairy products are all linked to healthy kidneys. Further consumption of magnesium, calcium, citrate, vegetables, and fruits can all result in a decreased risk of getting kidney stones.

The Trial on the Dash Diet to Determine the Effects of Sodium on Blood Pressure

The trial involved 412 adults, split into two groups: one group that followed the DASH diet and the other one that followed a normal American diet. Participants were given food and beverages that were enough to consume for one month (NIH, 2021). Their sodium daily intake was put at high, medium, and low. The high sodium intake group was given 3,300 mg of sodium per day, which is close to the American recommended daily intake. The medium group was given 2,300 mg, and the last group was given 1,500 mg.

The results of this study indicated that (NIH, 2021):

- Participants who had a lower amount of sodium intake had reduced blood pressure on both diets. However, the group that went through the DASH diet with reduced sodium of 1,500 mg had a lower blood pressure than the level of blood pressure that was found in the participants who were following the typical American diet for all three daily sodium levels.

- Cutting down on daily sodium intake reduced blood pressure for participants on both diets. However, the DASH diet in combination with the low sodium (1,500 mg or about half a teaspoon of salt) lowered blood pressure more than the typical American diet at all three daily sodium levels.

- Blood pressure decreased with each level of sodium reduction.

- Following the DASH diet, coupled with sodium reduction, lowers blood pressure better than only going on a DASH diet or reducing sodium intake.

- Both man and man showed they benefited from a lower sodium DASH diet, whether they had hypertension or not.

In a follow-up report, it was found that a combination of a DASH diet and reduced sodium helped people who had blood pressure levels that were considered above normal. The report also indicated that it's the individuals who started with the highest blood pressure had the most benefits (NIH, 2021).

Disadvantages of a DASH Diet

- **This diet requires every individual following it to plan their meals according to the servings allowed specifically for them.** If you are not used to cooking and meal planning, you may want some advice and guidance.

- **We have certain foods in this diet that are not in categories, like, for instance, avocado.** It becomes difficult to know which category they belong to, whether they are classified as fruits or a fat serving. Other foods are classified into categories that are not known to be correct or questionable. Another example is that of pretzels, which are classified together with grains despite having fewer nutrients and no fiber. Classifying frozen yogurt and dairy can also be questionable since most brands have very little calcium and vitamin D, and they contain high amounts of added sugar. Grains are all labeled as cereals, without considering that they can vary in nutrient and sugar content.

- **The diet may not be considered allergy-friendly.** Individuals with allergies and those who don't take lactose could be required to alter their meals and include other foods that are lactose-free.

- **There is a possibility of experiencing gas and bloating during the initial stages of the diet because of the high amounts of fiber from fruits, vegetables, and whole grains.** You can reduce the amount of fiber by only serving them once or twice a week, instead of every day.

- **It may be difficult to maintain this diet, especially for people who have been eating a typical American diet.** The DASH diet recommends that its followers must cut their sodium intake down to about 2,300 mg per day, and possibly further down to 1,500 mg per day. Most of the salt that is consumed on the usual American diet comes from processed foods, which are heavily restricted from the DASH diet (NIH, 2021). Most people can't just stop adding salt to their food, even if they don't eat processed foods.

- **The DASH diet does not recommend the consumption of convenience foods.** People might find it difficult to stick to this diet because there are appeal programs such as South Beach, Jenny Craig, and Weight Watchers. These weight loss programs allow people to subscribe to their services so that they get their meals delivered to their doorstep. The consumers simply receive the meals and snacks ready to eat, or they can just warm the goods in the microwave. This is what you can't enjoy with the DASH diet. Even going to a local market to get frozen ready-made meals will not be possible. This is one other setback because people may consider a DASH diet to be a lot of extra work.

- **The fact that there is no organized support for the DASH diet may be one disadvantage.** Other diet plans have support groups that can provide face-to-face guidance and counseling or peer-to-peer coaching. These support groups help people to stay motivated during certain times when they feel discouraged.

They also allow users to ask questions and learn new tips and tricks for their diets. This is one feature that is lacking in the DASH diet. However, if you are considering following this diet, don't be discouraged by this fact. Most of the registered dietitians know this diet very well and can assist you in developing the best meal plans. They can give you all the coaching and support that you need.

In this chapter, we have talked about the DASH diet, its meaning, and the types of people who can go for it, as well as those who can't. In Chapter 7, you're going to learn about intermittent fasting, what it focuses on, and who is suitable for it. We will also provide you with a list of the recommended foods in this diet, as well as its pros and cons.

Chapter 7:

Intermittent Fasting

Fasting, also known as intermittent fasting, provides us with an opportunity to actually get the best cells all the time and that's what we all need. —Steven Gundry

In the previous chapter, we discussed the DASH diet, how it works, and the food that's recommended to eat on this diet. The chapter has also touched on the people who are suitable for taking this diet. You have also learned about the advantages and disadvantages of eating the DASH diet. In this chapter, we are going to look at intermittent fasting, its definition, and the different methods of fasting that are available to us. We will also talk about the group of people that is recommended to go on this diet, as well as its advantages and disadvantages.

Intermittent fasting is one of the most popular diets in the United States. Besides being followed by a lot of people, this is a diet that is quite effective. This is a very easy diet to follow, which will significantly help you with weight loss, and it does wonders for your health.

Definition of Intermittent Fasting

Intermittent fasting refers to a meal timing schedule where the followers choose times to fast voluntarily and times to eat for a certain period. "Fasting" means going for a long time without eating, which is where the word "breakfast" originated from. When we sleep during the night, we don't eat and that's fasting. Our first meal in the morning has got to break this fast, hence the word *breakfast.*

If you have been through a situation where you don't have to eat for blood tests until the following day, this is the same concept with intermittent fasting. You just have to stop eating for a given period of time, but, on this diet, you have to do it on a regular basis. You may fast only during certain days, some days you eat as you normally would, and some days you have only one meal on schedule.

When you are fasting, you can only drink water and other calorie-free beverages like black coffee or tea. When it's time to eat, don't include processed foods in your meals—and forget about doorstep food deliveries or making a quick run through the drive-thru. You can choose to consume nutritious foods, but you don't have to totally divert from your way of eating.

What Kinds of Food Can You Eat During Your Fasting Period?

When you begin fasting, you don't eat; however, when it's time to eat, you just eat the food that you normally would. However, you don't have to go crazy. Otherwise, you may not achieve your weight loss goal if a majority of your meals consist of junk foods, are high in calories, or are fried. The good thing about intermittent fasting is that it allows you to eat different kinds of foods. You will be able to share your nutritious meal with other relatives and your friends.

Some experts recommend that those who try intermittent fasting follow the Mediterranean diet only as a guide to what they can eat. You can form a great diet when you include leafy green vegetables, lean meat, and whole-grain foods. Various diets concentrate on *what* they have to eat while intermittent fasting focuses on *when* you have to eat. Our bodies are flexible and able to go for a considerably long time without food, making it possible to go hours with no food and some even going for days of fasting or longer periods.

This fasting has since been practiced by our ancestors during Prehistoric times. During hunter-gathering, people could go for long periods without food. This is when human bodies learn to thrive without food. They did not have an option, as it took them a long time to gather food items, such as nuts and berries, and hunt the game; therefore, meal times were quite spaced.

How Intermittent Fasting Works

So many methods are available to practice intermittent fasting, but all of them focus on giving yourself time to fast before eating. The idea is for the body to exhaust all its sugar storage, and then start to burn the fat to get energy to use. This type of eating is totally different from the eating patterns of most Americans who like eating throughout the day.

If you eat three meals a day, plus snacks, and you don't like to exercise, your body will simply use the energy from the food you eat and will not burn any stored fat. This will make you not lose weight, but rather gain more. Intermittent fasting, therefore, works by making use of the calories you consumed during your last meal for energy. When that energy is finished, you don't eat anything and your body starts to burn stored fat for you to get more energy.

Methods of Practicing Intermittent Fasting

How long can you endure hunger without eating? Let's look at the available options so that you can choose the one suitable for you:

Going for a 12-Hour Fasting

For this fasting period, you simply have to go for 12 consecutive hours without eating food every day—that's the rule. It's easy to go through this type of fasting, especially for beginners, because the fasting period is not that long. Most of these hours are at night, when you're already sleeping. You just have to finish off a few remaining hours in the morning; and when it's time to eat, you can still consume the same amount of calories per day. Here, you may choose to start your fasting at 6 p.m. and then end the next morning at 6 a.m.

A 16-Hour Fasting

This kind of fasting is called the Leangains diet, or the 16:8 method. You don't eat for 16 hours and can only eat within an 8-hour limited time. It's helpful to remember that, when following this fasting method, men will fast for 16 hours while women fast for 14 hours. One can start fasting at 8 p.m. and not eat until noon.

Two Days a Week Fasting

Those who go for this fasting method will consume the average amounts of healthy meals for up to five days and then cut on their calorie consumption for the remaining two days. Also known as the 5:2 diet, men following this method will consume 600 calories and women will be limited to 500 calories. This is not a two-consecutive-day type of fasting, as you will be allowed to separate your fasting days. One can choose to fast on Tuesday and Friday while keeping in mind that you must allow at least one non-fasting day between your fasting days.

The Alternate Day Fasting

This method has several ways to practice it and it includes fasting one day and not the other. Some people choose to have a full day of not touching any solid foods. However, some people will allow 500 calories a day on this same method. During their eating days, other people may choose to eat as much food as they want.

24-Hour Fasting per Week

This method of fasting is also referred to as the "Eat-Stop-Eat" diet, and it limits the consumption of food for 24 consecutive hours. This can be done by starting to fast during lunch up until the next day's lunchtime again, or from one breakfast time to another.

Individuals going for this method can drink tea, water, or any other calorie-free beverages during the fasting period. During eating days, this method allows followers to go back to their normal eating routine and there's no limit on the specific foods they can eat. This is a bit of a challenging method since other people can end up having a headache, feeling fatigued, or irritated.

A Warrior Diet

This is one extreme way of fasting. It involves 20 hours of fasting where you can eat very small amounts of fruits and vegetables. The period of eating is only four hours a day, and you will be recommended to eat a lot of vegetables, healthy fats, carbohydrates, and proteins.

Benefits of Intermittent Fasting

The intermittent fasting benefits can go beyond just burning fat. Any changes that occur in the metabolic system can also affect the entire body as well as the brain. Some of these benefits include a lean body and a healthy brain. This fasting diet can help reduce type 2 diabetes, inflammatory bowel syndrome, certain types of cancer, as well as heart diseases (Good Food Is Good Medicine, 2022).

Let's check out some of the benefits of Intermittent fasting:

- **Sharp thinking and memory:** Intermittent fasting can help adult humans boost their verbal memory.

- **Helps with heart health:** This type of eating can help with reduced blood pressure and maintaining a healthy heart.

- **Physical fitness:** This eating plan can help with the maintenance of muscles in young men.

- **Helps with type 2 diabetes and obesity:** Those with type 2 diabetes are capable of doing away with insulin therapy, but they have to do so under the supervision of their doctors.

Disadvantages of Intermittent Fasting

Is Intermittent fasting a safe way to lose weight and stay healthy? We have people who try to use intermittent fasting diets to reduce weight, while some of them do it to address certain illnesses like arthritis, high cholesterol, or irritable bowel syndrome. However, this diet may not be suitable for everyone. So, before trying it or any other diet, you should seek guidance from your healthcare provider.

There are certain people who must totally stay away from intermittent fasting (Good Food Is Good Medicine, 2022):

- Teenagers and all the children under the age of 18

- Breastfeeding and expecting mothers

- Patients of type 1 diabetes who are on medication and administering insulin. Type 2 diabetic patients have been shown to benefit from intermittent fasting. However, there are concerns that those with type 1 diabetes may have problems if they try it since they are taking insulin.

- Those who can't control their eating habits. Such people must first consult their doctors before going on this diet to avoid problems.

Individuals without the above conditions can try intermittent fasting and it can bring changes to their lifestyle. If you start having anxiety or headaches after starting this diet, quickly consult your doctor, as people react to this diet in different ways.

This chapter has taught us about intermittent fasting. We now know that it is not about what we eat, but rather when to eat. We have also learned the different methods of practicing intermittent fasting.

There are certain groups of people who are not allowed to do these fastings, and we also discussed the pros and cons of intermittent fasting. In Chapter 8, we are going to learn about the Flexitarian diet and how it works. We will explore the foods that this diet focuses on and what is not recommended. To find out what is good and what's lacking about this diet, let's go through Chapter 8 and find out.

Chapter 8:

The Flexitarian Diet

Whether it's the food we cook, how we live, or the way we love... Our story is one that's "mostly" plant-based in the kitchen and "mostly" delicious out. Now, pull up your chair at our table slightly, learn the way we do it and how you think you can do it too. I only don't plan to wait for the dessert. —Wink, Wink

In Chapter 7, you read about intermittent fasting, its definition, and the type of people who are recommended for it, as well as those who are recommended to avoid it. You now know the various methods of intermittent fasting, as well as their advantages and disadvantages. In this chapter, we are going to discuss the flexitarian diet and what it means to go on such a diet. We will also look at how this diet works, the food that it focuses on, as well as its pros and cons.

Are you hunting for a diet that doesn't have a lot of rules and restrictions on calorie and meat consumption? The flexitarian diet is here for you. This diet is a combination of two known diets, the vegan and the vegetarian diets. The name "flexitarian" is made out of two words, "flexible" and "vegetarian". This means that it's a flexible diet that includes vegetarian foods. The diet is flexible in the sense that you can still enjoy animal products in moderation; however, it is a bit more flexible than the strict vegan and vegetarian diets. This diet will recommend you to add plant foods to your diet, without completely cutting out meat and other animal products.

The flexitarian diet is the number 2 U.S.-ranked diet, following the Mediterranean diet, which is ranked number 1 (Streit, 2022). It's popular because it's a simple-to-follow healthy diet that also accommodates meat in its meals. If you are scared to go on a vegetarian diet because you don't want to totally miss out on eating meat, the flexitarian diet can allow you to enjoy that chicken burger that you crave. However, you always have to remember that you still have to limit the amount of meat that you consume.

Another good thing about this diet is that it's a long-term diet that can allow you to maintain your body weight for a long time. This is contrary to other diets that follow for a certain period and stop, and you start regaining the body weight again. In your mind, there is no hurry in finishing the diet so you start eating the food that you enjoy again. You will still be enjoying the foods you love, while, at the same time, eating healthy foods.

What Is the Flexitarian Diet?

This is a semi-vegetarian diet or an eating plan that focuses on mainly plant-based foods, at the same time permitting you to consume meat and other animal products in moderation. Since the diet doesn't have stringent rules, it's suitable for people who want to wait for a healthy diet and are willing to reduce the amount of meat that they include in their meals. The flexitarian diet encourages the following:

- Your diet must focus mainly on consuming food like whole grains, legumes, vegetables, and fruits.

- Concentrate more on consuming more plant-based protein.

- Not to fully punish yourself by not eating meat at all, be flexible and allow yourself to include meat and animal products in your meals.

- Try to eat plant-based foods in their natural forms and avoid eating highly processed foods.

- Restrict the consumption of sweets and added sugars.

Because of its flexibility, which talks more about what healthy foods you need to consume rather than concentrating on stopping people from wanting to wait, this diet just became a popular one. Let's now look at the list of foods that you can include in your flexitarian diet:

- Make sure you include protein such as legumes, soybeans, tofu, and lentils

- Add non-starchy vegetables, such as green beans, Brussels sprouts, carrots, bell peppers, and cauliflower

- Include more starchy vegetables, like sweet potatoes, corn, winter squash, and peas.

- Don't forget to eat more healthy fruits, such as oranges, apples, cherries, grapes, and berries.

- Your carbohydrates must come from mainly whole grains like farro, buckwheat, and quinoa

- Get your healthy fats from walnuts, cashews, almonds, flaxseed, avocados, chia seeds, coconut, and olives

- Use unsweetened milk produced from plants, such as coconut milk, almond milk, soy milk, and hemp milk.

- Add some healthy herbs, seasonings, and spices, which include cumin, turmeric, oregano, basil, ginger, thyme, and mint, to your meals.

- Allow also condiments into your meals, such as nutritional yeast, soy sauce, apple cider vinegar, and zero sugar added ketchup

- Drink healthy beverages such as coffee, still water, tea, and sparkling water

When you get to that time of incorporating the much-needed meat and animal products, you can include the following foods:

- Eggs that are produced by free-range or pasture-raised chickens

- Your poultry must also be pasture-raised or organic

- Eat only wild-caught fish

- Your meat must be grass-fed or from pasture-raised animals

- Include dairy products from pastured animals or the ones that are grass-fed

Foods to Minimize on the Flexitarian Diet

This diet encourages its followers to limit the amount of meat and animal products that they include in their meals. They need to also reduce highly processed foods, added sugar, and refined grains. They need to limit the consumption of foods like:

- Highly processed meats, especially those processed using very high temperatures such as bacon, bologna, and sausage

- Well-refined carbohydrates, such as white bread, croissants, bagels, and white rice

- Sweet things with added sugar, like cakes, candy, cookies, soda, and doughnuts

- Junk foods like chicken nuggets, milkshakes, fries, and burgers

Going on a flexitarian diet is not all about reducing the amount of meat that you consume, refined carbs, added sugars, and so on; it's more about including healthy foods in your diet.

Guidelines Around Meat Consumption in the Flexitarian Diet

The name of this diet says it all— is supposed to be flexible. However, you need guidance on which type of meat you should consume and how much of it. The amount of meat that you eat depends on what you want to achieve and your commitment level, but it should be between 9 and 28 ounces per week, while, at the same time, following your healthy eating plan (Streit, 2022). This is why this diet is popular, as it gives you the privilege to choose how much meat you want to cut down.

We have three primary stages of how we should do it in terms of the meat consumption pattern:

Stage 1

For beginners, it is advised to not consume meat two days per week. During this initial period, you should limit your meat consumption to less than 28 ounces per week, which is during the five days of meat consumption.

Stage 2

The more you get used to this diet and become familiar with eating more vegetables and fruits, you will have to concentrate on turning your diet into more of a vegetarian diet. This also requires limiting your meat consumption to 18 ounces per week.

Stage 3

Increase your days of eating a vegetarian diet to five days a week. You will only eat meat on the two remaining days but don't exceed nine ounces for those two days.

Benefits of Eating a Flexitarian Diet

There are various benefits that we get from following a flexitarian diet. It may be a bit difficult to assess the benefits of this diet since it doesn't have a clear definition; however, since the diet involves the consumption of more of a vegan and vegetarian diet, we can look at the benefits that are compiled for a semi-vegetarian diet. Let's look at those benefits:

Lower Risk of Heart Disease

Consuming foods that contain a lot of fiber and healthy fats can help with a healthy heart. Individuals eating a vegetarian diet and fish are at a lower risk of getting ischemic heart disease in comparison to those who consume a lot of meat. A vegetarian diet also contains antioxidants, which can lower blood pressure and levels of cholesterol.

Weight Management

Going for a flexitarian diet will also help you to manage your weight. You will be able to achieve this because the flexitarian diet encourages limiting calorie consumption as well as highly processed foods, and promotes eating plant-based foods that contain fewer calories. People who consume more of a plant-based diet are more likely to lose more weight than those who don't.

Reduced Diabetes

A lot of people struggle with type 2 diabetes worldwide. Consumption of a healthy diet that is predominantly plant-based can help to reduce and avoid suffering from this disease. This may be because plant-based diets involve eating a lot of fiber and reduces the consumption of added sugar and unhealthy fats, which will also reduce the risk of sugar diabetes.

Can Prevent Cancer

Consuming a highly nutritious diet that includes plant foods like legumes, vegetables, and fruits reduces your risk of getting cancer. This diet is overall associated with a lower risk of all types of cancer, particularly colorectal cancer. Therefore, adding more vegetarian foods and reducing processed foods and meat can lower your cancer risk.

Disadvantages of a Flexitarian Diet

Eating a flexitarian diet can lead to a healthy lifestyle; however, certain individuals can run short of other nutrients because of the limitations of meat and animal products. Watch out for nutrient deficiencies such as calcium, zinc, vitamin B12, iron, and omega-3 fatty acids. Vitamin B12 is only available in animal products; so, when you reduce the consumption of animal products, it means that you won't get enough of the vitamin (Streit, 2022).

The flexitarian diet contains nuts, whole grains, seeds, and legumes, which contain iron and zinc. You may need to add vitamin C to improve the absorption of this iron. Some people on this diet may choose to cut down on dairy products, which are a good source of calcium. This means they will have to replace them with plant-based sources to get enough of the calcium. Plants that can provide you with a lot of calcium include kale, sesame seeds, chad, and bok choy.

Followers of a flexitarian diet must also remember that they need to get enough omega-3 fatty acids, and we normally get them from fatty fish. Therefore, because there are limits to your fish consumption, you may need to supplement it with fish oil or algal oil to maintain the requirements.

What you need to remember is that a flexitarian diet can allow you to eat meat and animal products. If you plan your diet well and make sure it's balanced, you will not even have a problem with nutrient deficiencies.

In this chapter, we have discussed the flexitarian diet and why it is favored by many people. The next chapter is going to cover the Zone Diet, why we should eat it, and the types of foods that it focuses on. We will also look at the advantages and disadvantages of using the diet.

Chapter 9:

The Zone Diet

To be genetically correct, man needs a modern version of a Neo-Paleolithic diet, a diet that's based on his current genetic makeup. That's what is meant by Zone-A highly favorable diet: a diet that is consistent with humans' genetic structure, the one that has changed very slightly in the last 100,000 years. —Barry Sears

Chapter 8 has taken us through the flexitarian diet and why it is referred to as a "flexible diet." We also learned the types and sources of foods that are included in this diet. We now understand the benefits and setbacks associated with the flexitarian diet as well. In this chapter, we are going to read about the Zone Diet, its definition, and the types of foods that it promotes. We will also discuss what people like about this diet and why other people won't go for it. Everything is explained in this chapter, so let's continue reading.

The Zone Diet is one of the eating plans that aims to reduce inflammation, but it also focuses on reducing body weight loss. Having been created by Dr. Barry Sears, this diet has been around to help people for more than 30 years, helping its followers to shed excess pounds and get a good mental and physical performance. The Zone Diet involves a dietary program that is science-based and is meant to lessen the amount of inflammation in the body (Dr. Sears Zone, n.d.).

What Is the Zone?

This is something that can actually be clinically measured from your body. It is the physiological condition or state of your body at a particular time (Dr. Sears Zone, n.d.). When one is said to be "in the zone," they have optimized their ability to manage diet-induced inflammation.

Having some inflammation results in you gaining weight, aging quicker, or becoming sick. The tricky part of the diet is that, as long as inflammation is reduced in your body, you will be able to lessen the amount of fat in your body at a faster rate, be able to reduce chronic illnesses, and age at a slower rate.

Definition of the Zone Diet

The Zone Diet is an eating plan that is aimed at reducing body inflammation, as well as reducing weight. It encourages its followers to eat unsaturated fats and antioxidants, which include omega-3 fatty acids and a supplement of polyphenol antioxidants. The Zone Diet also limits calorie consumption, however, it doesn't specify how much in terms of quantity must be consumed. This is one diet that restricts people's eating to particular ratios of 30% protein, 20% fats, and 40% carbohydrates (Dr. Sears Zone, n.d.). Part of this diet requires carbs with a low glycemic index, which is when they release fewer amounts of sugar into your bloodstream so that you stay nourished for a longer period.

This diet encourages people to eat protein from skinless chicken, low-fat dairy, fish, tofu, egg whites, soy, turkey, and other meat substitutes. When choosing carbohydrates, followers of this diet are encouraged to choose carbs that are low on the glycemic index (GI), which is a level of rankings on how carbs impact blood sugar.

Eating low GI carbs makes you feel fuller for a long amount of time, maintains your metabolism, and steadies your blood sugar. Bad carbohydrates, or high-GI carbs, will simply do the opposite. The targeted sources are non-starchy vegetables that exclude corn, peas, and fruits (but not bananas and raisins). You can also eat oatmeal and barley. Try to avoid starchy foods like pasta, cereals, bagels, bread, and potatoes.

Although small amounts of unsaturated fats can be added, stay away from fatty red meat, liver, and egg yolks, as well as any organ meat, as they contain high amounts of saturated fats. To measure the quantity of meat that you can eat, simply use your palm. A proper portion of meat will fit inside your palm without overlapping. For women, this will give you 3 ounces and men will get 4 ounces.

Also, take note of your eating times, as followers of the Zone Diet must value their meal and snack times. If you fail to eat at the right times, your blood sugar will go down, causing you to have hunger pangs. Your eating times should be within a five-hour limit, so don't exceed these hours without eating something. Eat your breakfast as soon as you wake up, but don't spend an hour without eating your breakfast from the time you wake up. Let's say you eat your breakfast at 7 a.m., your lunch should be at 12 noon, then you will have a snack at 5, eat your dinner at 7 p.m., and then have another snack at 11 p.m.

The following rules must be obeyed when following the Zone Diet:

- You must have something to eat within one hour of waking up.

- Every meal should start with a low-fat protein, after that, you can eat low GI carbohydrates and healthy fats.

- Create a habit of eating small but more frequent meals during the day. Consider eating meals every 4-6 hours and 2-2.5 hours from the time you had a snack, even if you don't feel hungry.

- Eat a lot of omega-3 fatty acids as well as polyphenols, since they help reduce inflammation.

- Drink lots of water, as it's recommended to drink at least 8 medium-sized glasses of water a day.

When it comes to carbohydrates, choose carbs that come from fruits and vegetables. Avoid starchy foods and go for foods with a low GI. These foods stay in your stomach longer before being completely digested, which will help reduce blood sugar spikes after meals. Allow carbohydrates to make up two-thirds of your meals or snacks. Try to avoid eating saturated fats and replace them with healthy fats, such as olive oil, avocado, and nuts.

Also, make sure to include polyphenols, which are a type of antioxidant. These will assist your body to neutralize free radicals, which can cause cell damage and, eventually, can cause cancer. Eating vegetables and fruits can help provide plenty of antioxidants.

Omega-3 is also good for your health, as it can help minimize inflammation in your body. Sources of omega-3 fatty acids include sardines and oily fish. Followers of the Zone Diet must check the level of their hunger before meals; if they don't feel hungry and have a clear mind, then they are considered to be in "the zone."

When following the Zone Diet, individuals should eat a balanced diet following the recommendations:

- Proteins must only make one-third of the meal

- Include two-thirds of carbohydrates

- A small amount of unsaturated fats

Your protein must come from fish, poultry, beef, low-fat dairy products, beans, lentils, guys, seeds, eggs, and tofu.

The sources of carbohydrates must include fruits and non-starchy vegetables like spinach, broccoli, green beans, mushrooms, and asparagus. You can also include oatmeal, barley, and pulses, such as lentils and beans.

Avoid sources of carbohydrates such as sweets, energy drinks, baked foods, breads (especially white bread), rice, pasta, and starchy vegetables like peas, squash, potatoes, and corn.

Advantages of a Zone Diet

- **Good nutritional value:** The food portions from each food group generally follow the required guidelines: a bigger portion of carbohydrates, a smaller portion of proteins, and little fats. People are encouraged to eat lean meat and lots of fruits and vegetables. Unhealthy foods like sweets, chips, and sugary drinks are not recommended.

- **It's a flexible diet:** This is a flexible diet because it allows a variety of foods to be consumed. It also encourages the consumption of 3 meals per day, all of them being almost the same size, which is close to normal-sized meals that people usually eat. There is not much of a change and people find the planning of the meals to be quite easy.

- **Healthy choice of protein sources:** The Zone Diet recommends people eat protein that comes from healthy sources, such as lean meat, low-fat dairy products, tofu, and egg whites. Unsaturated fats are encouraged, and higher-fat meats are consumed in less quantities. Eating higher protein foods can help to avoid muscle loss and make you feel fuller for a longer amount of time, as well as help to burn calories.

What Are the Setbacks of This Diet?

This diet may be difficult to sustain since there are specific portions for each meal component. Some people may find it hard to know the exact quantities of protein, carbohydrates, and fats that will make the meal "Zone Diet approved" when they are not eating homemade meals. Certain individuals might find the diet depriving of other foods, which can make them reluctant to get committed to the diet.

- Besides the Zone Diet being encouraged to help with certain chronic illnesses such as diabetes, heart and cancer, patients with these diseases must first consult their healthcare providers before they choose to go for it.

- This diet may also be complicated to track. Other diets have one thing to track, maybe fats, carbs, or proteins. This is not the case with the Zone Diet, where you have to count fats, proteins, and carbs all at once, which might be inconvenient for some people.

We have gone through the Zone Diet and what it means to follow such a diet. In Chapter 10, we are going to look at the Weight Watchers diet and how it works. You will read about the advantages and disadvantages of the Weight Watchers diet, as we also discuss what the point system means.

Chapter 10:

The Weight Watchers

The food you eat can be either the safe an most powerful medicine or the slowest poison. —Sukhraj S. Dhillon

We have already covered the Zone Diet in the last chapter. So, now that you understand the foods that you can eat on this diet, it's up to you to make it one of your favorites or not since you also understand its benefits and downsides.

In this chapter, you are going to learn about the Weight Watchers diet, its definitions, and how it works. You will also read about its advantages and disadvantages. The Weight Watchers diet is one of the highest followed diets, gaining the highest approval votes by doctors, putting it number 1 in 2020 (Shoemaker, 2022). This is the reason why even celebrities like Oprah Winfrey are following this diet.

Definition of the Weight Watchers Diet

The Weight Watchers site, also referred to as WW, can be described as a weight management program that deals with individual points with regard to factors such as a person's height, weight, or age. This information is used to give points, which are then used to determine and track the amount of food consumed and recommend them to eat a healthy diet.

This personalized meal plan is quite flexible, permitting its followers to have a choice of a variety of foods, while, at the same time, being able to use points to track their intake. Support groups are available for this diet, allowing those on the diet to meet and get support to remain motivated. Followers of this diet go for weekly meetings, which other diets don't do. The program promotes a long-term healthy lifestyle and overall well-being.

As for the answer to the question of whether the WW helps people to lose weight: yes, it helps people manage their weight. The fact that the diet recommends its followers to consume fewer calories than the one they use is a clear recipe for losing weight. It's a diet that is simple to follow, promotes the condition of nutrient-dense foods, and avoids unhealthy foods such as fried foods and sweet foods with added sugar and calories—which can make you lose a lot of points. It is alleged that followers of the WW diet lose weight two times faster than they could have lost with a traditional diet alone (Shoemaker, 2022). It is the support meetings and encouragement from the WW program that push people to lose more weight.

Advantages of the WW Program

Offers Individual Choices

Unlike other diets that talk of one-size-fits-all diets, which are not, in fact, suitable for everyone, the WW program deals with individual needs. The points system that is used in this program makes people choose what they want to eat and make the quantities that are suitable for their needs. If you are allowed to eat what you want on a diet, that will make you more willing to stick to the diet. The WW continues to implement more new ideas to change which bring flexibility to the diet.

Provides Lifelong Skills

Most provided diets are just for the short term, which is opposite to the WW program. It educates people on measuring their food portions, which can still be helpful to you even after stopping the diet. The tracking system, as it tracks your food intake, will also help with long-term weight management.

The moment we measure the food portions that we eat, we already manage the amount of food that we consume. The most important thing to bear in mind is that the bigger portions must come from lower energy-dense foods and smaller portions come from high-energy foods. This will ensure weight loss as well as weight management. This program also supplies its followers with eating tips, recipes, and advice, which allows them to make healthy meals from home.

No Total Prohibition of Any Food

Foods that are prohibited can lead to an uncontrolled way of eating, such as binge eating. There is a tendency for people struggling to totally do away with certain foods; however, when you tell yourself that you are not allowed to consume this good, the more you start to crave that food. Allowing yourself to eat a variety of foods will help you to have control over your eating habits. When off-limit foods are put on the table during family meals, especially desserts, children will end up eating smaller quantities of food than usual. Rather than stating the foods that are allowed to eat or not, the Weight Watchers diet provides Fit Points, which can help you to get more personal points.

No Abrupt Weight Loss

Quick-fix diets are not good, as some people will end up losing shape or having sagging stomachs when they use alternative methods to lose weight. The WW diet recommends losing 1-2 pounds every week, which is also recommended by the National Institute of Health. This diet encourages gradual weight loss to give your body time to gain the shape that you want while you're losing weight.

Losing weight very fast can make you regain that weight in the near future. If you are willing to lose weight in a slow and steady manner, look no further than the WW diet. This diet goes with you slowly as your body adjusts to the new way of eating.

Enough Support Is Available

The WW diet provides a lot of support to its followers through online support groups, virtual coaches, and one-on-one support, as well as community support that allows only members to attend and is available at all times. This has been seen to significantly improve the success of those using the diet.

The program also has a lot of recipes as well as workout programs that are a part of the membership benefits. This diet uses a barcode that is used for tracking the meals and you will be able to create new recipes and serve them as well.

Good Exercise Programs

Same as the National Institute of Health, which recommends food exercises, the WW diet also promotes exercise. The NIH states that adult individuals between the ages of 18 and 64 should be engaged in average-vigorous physical aerobic activities for at least 150 minutes per week (Shoemaker, 2022). Alternatively, they can do 75 minutes of vigorous aerobic workouts within a week. On top of this, it also encourages muscle-strengthening exercises for at least two days per week.

The WW eating plan encourages its followers to create activity goals that they can follow, either daily or weekly. You will then be required to add any extra activities, which will make you earn extra personal points on each workout added to your normal weekly schedule. Here, you are given the freedom to choose the workouts that you like and do them. Your WW membership workout schedule also includes cardiovascular workouts that are led by an instructor, yoga, core, pilates, as well as stretching workouts.

Disadvantages of the WW Diet

Besides the WW being a diet with a variety of benefits, it has its own shortfalls. Let's go through these pitfalls and see how bad they are:

It May Be Costly to Follow This Diet

It is important to take note of the cost of the WW membership plan before you can start considering joining it. You need to choose the duration that will suit your pocket, all while considering the amount of work that you need to achieve your goal weight and body.

The packages range from 1 month, 3 months, or 6 months, and then, going forward, you will have a leeway to select and add one of your choices. These choices include workouts that are led by an instructor or one-on-one coaching, where you are required to pay an extra amount.

Make sure you choose the duration that you will be able to achieve and pay for every month, while also making sure that you stay within your budget. If you try and pay your fees in advance, you may get a considerable discount. You could also consult your insurance provider and see what they have to offer. Most of the insurance providers can offer a good discount, and some can even pay you back your money if you are working with Weight Watchers.

Point System May Be Tedious for Some

Some people are not comfortable with the system of counting points at the same time as they track their nutrition. Maintaining your points on a daily basis can be stressful, and it may also be difficult for certain people to stick to what they are recommended to eat for the whole day. This may lead to unhealthy behavior toward food, and result in uncontrolled eating patterns.

Chapter 10 has covered the Weight Watchers eating plan and what it means to follow this diet. In the next chapter, you will learn about the harmonious diet, and what it means to have such a diet.

Chapter 11:

Creating the Harmonious Diet

A person cannot think properly, love genuinely, or sleep nicely, if one has not eaten well. —Virginia Woolf

Chapter 10 has taken us through the Weight Watchers diet, its definitions, and how it works. We also learned about the foods that are recommended to eat on this diet, as well as its pros and cons. This chapter is going to concentrate on the harmonious diet and how it's created. We're also going to analyze the strengths and weaknesses of each diet. In this chapter, we will read about how a variety of diets can be combined to form a diet that is balanced.

The way you dine is just as important as the type of food that you eat. This can affect the way we feel. If you notice that the food makes you feel fatigued or anxious after eating it, it's not really good for you. This type of food is likely to be toxic to your body, like, for instance, highly refined foods. The same feeling can happen if you eat a large meal that consists of basically highly processed carbohydrates, potatoes, rice, or bread. This is because high-energy foods can lead to a spike in your sugar levels, causing a likely fluctuation in hormones, as well as brain neurotransmitters, that can change your mood and the way you feel.

For you to feel good after consuming a meal, you must eat healthy foods and a balanced meal. There is a need for you to eat harmoniously and consume foods that are nutrient-dense and full of life. Try to avoid foods that have been overcooked, irradiated, or pasteurized because they lose their nutritional value during the cooking process.

It is advised to add foods that contain healthy unsaturated fats like seeds, nuts, olive oil, avocado, and coconut oil to your diet. These types of food are needed for a healthy nervous system. Go for only organic foods and consume a variety of colored vegetables, leafy greens, and fruits. Such foods will help with digestion, as well as detoxify the body. When a body fails to receive the much-needed nutrients, it will end up dysfunctional as your body tries to compensate for these nutrients. Lack of these food requirements can lead to brain fog, poor digestion, and fatigue.

Eating Harmoniously

When we talk of eating harmoniously, we refer to the nature of the environment where you eat your food from. Find a suitable place at home, where everyone will be sitting down. You must be able to pay attention to eating and focus on chewing your food. Avoid working during meals or having something that makes noise and draws your attention, like a TV. Also, try to avoid using your cell phone or any other electronic device.

What Are the Strengths and Weaknesses of Every Diet

All the diets that we have discussed have their own type of foods that are believed to provide a significant change toward weight loss and health provision. In addition to these strengths, you find out that there are shortfalls as well. Let's look at what each diet is strong at and where it's lacking.

The Mediterranean Diet

This diet is usually prescribed by doctors to patients who suffer from chronic illnesses like high blood pressure and heart disease. One advantage of eating a Mediterranean diet is that it does not totally exclude any food group, as it promotes the use of various nutrient-dense foods. This means you can still enjoy the flavors of different types of foods while, at the same time, getting the required amount of nutrients that you need.

As for the weaknesses of the Mediterranean diet, there are a few notable ones. For instance, although it doesn't include high-cost branded foods or even expensive special supplements, many consumers complain about the cost of certain items like olive oil, nuts, seeds, and fish. If you scrutinize the price of seafood, it looks more expensive than other protein foods. But, you have to remember that there are various ways to shop on a budget, inclusive of seafood.

The Keto Diet

The aim of the keto diet is to push your body to use fat for energy instead of using the usual glucose. When your body fails to get the required glucose, it goes into a ketosis state. In the beginning, this diet was prescribed to treat childhood epilepsy; however, it has recently started to be used for weight loss.

One of the biggest disadvantages of this diet is that sometimes your appetite or food cravings might mess with your eagerness to lose weight. Feeling hungry when you are trying to lose weight may be the biggest stumbling block to achieving your goals. This is what makes a lot of people give up and start to eat their normal traditional diet again.

The biggest weakness of the Keto diet is dehydration. A keto diet can result in the loss of water before the person can even start to lose fat. Therefore, when starting to follow this diet, the first side effect that you will experience is dehydration. You will feel dehydrated when your body loses too much fluids, which means you will be losing fluids at a faster rate than you can take in. Signs and symptoms of dehydration include dry mouth or throat, passing dark-colored urine, tiredness, dizziness, and always feeling thirsty.

The Plant-Based Diet

Following a plant-based diet helps you lose weight and have a leaner and manageable body. It becomes easier for you to engage in any type of sporting activity than someone who is on a diet. Because the diet is filled with more dietary fiber, you can eat more without having to significantly increase your amount of calorie intake.

The biggest weakness of the plant-based diet is that it may be difficult for you to make a well-balanced whole plant-based meal, particularly if you are on a strict vegetarian or vegan diet. It may be challenging to know what nutrients are making up your meal unless you carefully plan these meals, maybe with the help of a dietician. If you fail to do this, you may not be able to meet your daily protein requirements.

The Paleolithic Diet

The biggest strength of the Paleolithic diet is that it's accepted by our DNA. It requires you to cut down on processed foods and added sugars and focus on whole foods, which are the foods that our bodies are ready to eat and digest without problems.

The weakness of the Paleolithic diet is that there is a fear that individuals following the diet might run short of certain nutrients like vitamins, fiber, and other key nutrients. Failure to consume food like whole grains, legumes, and dairy products means that you may have deficiencies in nutrients such as vitamin B, vitamin D, and calcium. When you continue lacking these nutrients, this can put you at risk of suffering from osteoporosis.

The DASH Diet

The DASH diet recommends people eat foods that are easy to access and found in most food stores. The strength of this diet is that all the foods on the list are not hard-to-get ingredients, foods, subscriptions, or supplements for those on the program. For this diet, you can find everything you want to know about it online, where it is free of charge, which may not be the same as other diet plans.

The weaker part of this diet is that it needs every individual following it to plan their meals according to the servings allowed specifically for them. If you are not used to cooking and meal planning, you may want some advice and guidance.

Intermittent Fasting

Intermittent fasting is great for burning fat, providing sharp thinking and good memory. It can also help adults to boost their verbal memory. There are certain people who must avoid intermittent fasting, which is the biggest weakness of this diet. People like teenagers and all children under the age of 18, breastfeeding and expecting mothers, and patients with type 1 diabetes who are on medication and administering insulin cannot go on this diet.

The Flexitarian Diet

This is a diet that is quite flexible. It has a lot of followers because it doesn't totally prohibit the consumption of meat and animal products, but rather allows people to eat them in moderation.

One weakness of this diet is that certain individuals can run short of other nutrients because of the limitations of meat and animal products. Watch out for nutrient deficiencies such as calcium, zinc, vitamin B12, iron, and omega-3 fatty acids. Vitamin B12 is only available in animal products, so when you reduce the consumption of animal products, it will mean you won't get enough of the vitamin.

The Zone Diet

The Zone Diet's strength is that food portions from each food group generally follow the required guideline, which is a bigger portion of carbohydrates, smaller portions of proteins, and little fats. People are encouraged to eat lean meat and a lot of fruits and vegetables. Unhealthy foods like sweets, chips, and sugary drinks are not recommended.

One weakness of this diet is that it may be difficult to sustain since there are specific portions for each meal component. Some people can find it hard to know the exact quantities of protein, carbohydrates, and fats that will make the meal, particularly when they are not homemade meals. Certain individuals might find the diet depriving of other foods, which can make them reluctant to get committed to the diet.

The Weight Watchers Diet

The strength of this diet, unlike other diets that talk of one-size-fits-all programs, is that the WW program deals with individual needs. The points system that is used in this program makes people choose what they want to eat and make the quantities that are suitable for their needs. If you are allowed to eat what you want on a diet, that will make you more willing to stick to the diet. The WW continues to implement more new ideas to change, which brings flexibility to the diet.

The weakness of this diet is the cost of the WW membership plan, which you need to take note of before you start to consider joining it. You need to choose the duration that will suit your pocket, while, at the same time, considering the amount of work that you need to achieve on your body. The packages may start from 1 month, 3 months, or 6 months. Then, going forward, you will have a leeway to select and add one of your choices, such as the workouts, which are led by an instructor, or one-on-one coaching, where you are required to pay an extra amount.

Crafting a Balanced, Sustainable Combination Diet

The harmonious food combining program is not there to only make you lose weight, but rather to encourage you to eat harmoniously, considering the needs of your digestive system. On top of that, you will also lose weight because of the healthy foods that you eat such as fruits, vegetables, wholesome nuts, and fish, as highly processed foods are prohibited. Using this diet can do wonders for individuals with digestive problems; and you are most likely going to have a flat tummy, decreased baseline, and a good skin complexion, as well as regular movement of the bowl.

The food that we have, especially in its natural forms like avocado, contains all the nutrients found in the three food groups that we have: carbohydrates, protein, and fats. Grains contain about 10% protein, and it's not as high in concentration as what we find in meat.

Harmonious Food Combining Groups

The Harmonious Food combining program values four primary groups, which are starch, protein, fruits, and neutral.

- The sources of concentrated protein are mainly meat, eggs, fish, and dairy products

- Starches are also concentrated in foods such as cereals, grains, and starchy vegetables, which are energy-giving foods.

- Other nutrients, such as alkaline-creating foods and fats, belong to the neutral group. These types of food include dairy fat, butter, some fruits, and vegetables.

- In the fruits category, we have sweet, acidic, and sub-acidic fruits. When eating fruits from these different categories, it is advised not to mix them and make sure that when you want watermelon, you eat it alone. Foods that form alkaline can be consumed in combination with yogurt, nuts, or kefir. You can use sweet fruits to sweeten meals, especially when they are cooked.

Rules for Harmonious Food Combinations

- The combination of foods from the starch and protein groups is not supposed to be combined during mealtime.

- It is recommended to combine foods from the neutral group with starchy foods or protein.

- You are advised to have one starch meal and one protein meal per day.

- Fruits must be consumed alone, especially during breakfast times.

- There must be a gap of about four hours between meals, and at least two hours after eating fruits.

In this chapter, we have covered the harmonious diet, what it means to try it, as well as the kinds of foods that are consumed during the diet. In the next chapter, we are going to discuss the implementation of the harmonious diet and how you can smoothly move to using this diet.

Chapter 12:

Executing the Harmonious Diet

In Chapter 11, we discussed the harmonious diet, so you now know what it means to eat harmoniously. We have also looked at what we can take from other diets to create a harmonious diet. You have also read about the strengths and weaknesses of all the other diets. This chapter is going to focus on ideas and tips for moving to a harmonious diet, how to plan meals, and strategies that you can use to keep a sustainable way of eating.

Eating a healthy diet in life is good for the protection against malnutrition and chronic illnesses such as stroke, heart disease, cancer, and type 2 diabetes. Lack of exercise, together with unhealthy diets, are the leading causes of poor health and illnesses throughout the world. Let's look at the foods that we can use to make a combination diet that helps people with weight management and a higher life expectancy.

Fresh Vegetables and Fruits

If you manage to consume at least 400g from five different types of fruits and vegetables each day, you help yourself to reduce the risk of getting non-communicable diseases (CDs) and you get an adequate supply of dietary fiber. You can improve your consumption of fruits and vegetables by doing the following:

- Make sure you add enough vegetables every time you prepare your meals

- Consume healthy raw fruits and vegetables when you it's time to have a snack

- Look for the fruits and vegetables that are in season and make them part of your daily meals

- Get a habit of consuming a variety of dark-colored vegetables and fruits.

Fat Consumption

It's always a good move to reduce the amount of fat that you eat to not more than 30% of your total energy consumption. This is crucial for body weight maintenance. You can again reduce the risk of having noncommunicable diseases by doing the following:

- Maintaining your consumption of saturated fats to not more than 10% of your total energy intake per day

- Make sure you avoid eating saturated and trans-fats and eat unsaturated fats

- Your daily consumption of trans-fats should not exceed 1% of the total energy consumption

If you want to minimize the amount of your trans-fat and saturated-fat intake, you should:

- **Use cooking methods that don't require a lot of fat when cooking your food.** For example, try boiling or steaming your vegetables instead of frying them.

- **Avoid using lard, butter, or ghee to prepare your meals.** Try to replace these fats with unsaturated fats like sunflower, canola, safflower, or corn oil.

- **Make sure you eat low-fat dairy products and lean meat.** Remember to remove all visible fat from your meat before cooking it.

- **Stay away from eating fried foods, baked, and already-packed foods and snacks.** Items like pies, cookies, cakes, wafers, and doughnuts are all prepared using trans-fats.

Sodium and Potassium Intake

Consuming a lot of sodium and inadequate potassium intake can lead to increased high blood pressure which leads to a risk of stroke and heart diseases. Recommended daily sodium intake is less than 5g daily, but people just consume a lot of salt not even knowing how much they are consuming per day.

You can reduce your sodium intake by:

- Adding small amounts of salt to your food when cooking

- Not bringing salt or high-sodium sauces to the table during meal times

- Reducing the consumption of snacks with too much salt

- Choosing foods and ingredients with lower sodium content

Sugars

A total of 10% limit of sugar consumption must always be kept in mind, although reducing it to at least 5% will help with additional health benefits. The consumption of free sugars can cause people to have tooth decay. Eating high-calorie foods that are high in free sugars can lead to weight gain, which can cause obesity. To minimize your sugar intake you should:

- Reduce the amounts of food that contain high quantities of sugar such as sweets, snacks, and beverages with added sugars

- Consume raw vegetables and fruits during snacking time

Harmonious Meal Planning and Recipes

The following is a guide to how you can plan your harmonious meals:

Example 1

- **Breakfast alkaline:** Serve your breakfast with tea or coffee, accompanied by a fruit salad. For your mid-morning snack, you can make for yourself an oaty bar or just eat nuts.

- **Starchy lunch:** For your lunch meal, you can eat some vegetable stew, served with rice or potatoes. You can also have a lunch of vegetable soup served with wholesome bread or just serve a smoked salmon sandwich. You can add a salad to your lunch meal using onion, lettuce, tomato, and radishes. For your afternoon fruit snack, you can eat a banana.

- **Protein dinner:** Your dinner must mainly consist of protein. Serve yourself some grilled fish or meat in combination with a vegetable mash, grilled vegetables, and a salad.

Example 2

- **Starchy breakfast:** For your starchy breakfast, you can have toast served with honey or porridge. You can also choose to serve a healthy oat cake with coffee or tea. Eat celery sticks for the mid-morning snack or you can simply eat nuts.

- **Alkaline lunch:** For your alkaline lunch, you can choose to have herb tea, coffee, or tea, along with a vegetable salad served with mixer leaves. For your afternoon snack, you can have some fruit pieces.

- **Protein dinner:** Serve some baked meat with mashed root vegetables, and you can also add a mixed salad. Wine can also be served as a drink, but it's optional.

Tips for Maintaining a Long-term Balanced Diet

Every person has the ability to positively contribute to this world. You have the responsibility to implement a healthy diet that makes a difference in your life and for other people. Here are some of the foods that can improve your health:

- **Include more fruits and vegetables in your diet:** Eating more fruits and vegetables can improve your health and does not have any negative impact on the environment. We also have fruits and vegetables that need to be consumed less frequently since they require a lot of resources to transport them, as they are fragile or need refrigeration. These may include berries, hot house cucumbers, tomatoes, mange-touts, and green beans that are imported from the Southern Hemisphere.

- **Eat plenty of fruits and vegetables that are in season:** These are more sustainable as they will be found locally.

- **Avoid overconsumption:** Don't consume more than what is required, particularly treats.

- **Watch your fats:** Replace animal fat with plant-based fats, with olive oil being your best option.

- **Avoid eating highly refined cereals and go for whole grains:** Whole grains don't require a lot of resources for processing. Some of these foods may include whole-grain pasta, quinoa, whole-wheat bread, as well as brown rice.

In this chapter, we have learned about how you can implement a harmonious diet, meal plans, and strategies for having a long-lasting sustainable diet. In the next chapter, we will wrap the entire book up, leaving you with a delightful summary that you can sink your teeth into.

Conclusion

This book is the road to a healthy lifestyle. The diets provided are available for you to choose from so that you can eat foods that keep you away from certain chronic diseases. Consuming food without following any guidelines, as well as poor exercise, can lead to a sedentary lifestyle and, possibly, a lower life expectancy. Give yourself time to go through this book, read all the diets provided, and choose the one that is suitable for you and the lifestyle you want to live.

Nobody will say they can't have any suitable diet for themselves because the diets provided are there to satisfy everyone's needs. Those who don't want to eat meat can choose to go for the vegan or the vegetarian diet. We also have a group of people who don't want to miss meat at all but want to consume it in moderation and can follow a flexitarian diet. The Mediterranean diet is there for the provision of a balanced diet and one that will help you lose weight at the same time.

We have individuals who struggle with good absorption and find it difficult to consume modern diets. This makes the Paleolithic diet the best choice since it is easily accepted by our DNA and it's a meal that was trusted by our ancestors. Those who are not comfortable following a one-size-fits-all type of diet are advised to follow the Weight Watchers diet. This program provides meals that satisfy individual needs so you eat the quantities suitable for only you. This diet provides a lot of support, starting from online support to community support.

The harmonious diet is also available for those who want to eat healthy foods in a satisfying way. The diet helps us to lose weight and stay healthy. This diet also provides less damage to the environment as it encourages the consumption of fruits and vegetables. Knowing how to combine foods in this diet is one key to eating healthy meals.

What we simply have to remember is that the foods that are available for us to consume these days are no longer the same. These highly processed foods, canned, and sugary drinks are the root cause of our problems. At times, we feel we don't have time to prepare healthy meals and find it easier to just order a pizza or rush through the drive-thru. But, keep in mind that some foods are excellent to the taste when they aren't good for your body.

Now, the choice of whether you want a change or not is yours. If you want to live a healthy life, then go ahead, choose a diet, and see how many benefits you will receive from changing the way you eat. You will enjoy a slim body, a life that has a reduced risk of getting non-communicable diseases, and an increase in your life expectancy. Love starts by loving yourself. You can't love anything or anyone in this world if you don't love yourself first. Bring a change in this world, and bring love for yourself and others too through leading a healthy lifestyle.

Appendix :

Sample Meal Plans

Get started on the right foot for the harmonious diet through the use of these helpful meal plans and recipes. This book will equip you with the necessary knowledge for you to understand the dietary choices that Americans can select from. The best elements of each diet can be put together to form a more sustainable nutritional diet. Below are three meal plans for each meal time and snack, using the diet principles for breakfast, lunch, dinner, and snacks.

Breakfast Meals

The Harmonious Breakfast Bowl

Ingredients:

- Yogurt (Greek)

- Mixed berries, which can be blueberries, raspberries, or strawberries

- Well-chopped walnuts or almonds

- Optional: honey

Directions:

- Put a good amount of yogurt inside your mixing bowl

- Top it up with different types of berries and chopped nuts

- Drizzle some honey, if needed

Avocado With Egg Breakfast Sandwich

Ingredients:

- Full-grain English muffin

- Nicely-mashed avocado

- Egg (poached)

- Sliced tomato

- Clean leaves of spinach

Directions:

- First, toast your English muffin

- On one side of the muffin, spread your crushed avocado. On the other side, place your spinach and the slices of tomato

- Add your poached egg and then make it into a sandwich

Mushroom Spinach Omelet

Ingredients:

- Sliced mushrooms

- Eggs

- Cleaned leaves of spinach

- Olive oil

- Optional: feta cheese

Directions:

- Put a bit of olive oil in a frying pan and add spinach when oil is warm

- Add mushrooms and fry until they look tender

- Beat the egg and add it to the pan

- Cook until the mixture is set, then fold it into half

- You can add feta cheese if prefer

Full-grain and Nut Butter Pancakes

Ingredients:

- Pancake mix (whole-grain)

- Cashew or almond nut butter

- Bananas (sliced)

- Optional: syrup, (preferably maple)

Directions:

- Make your pancakes following the directions given on the package

- Apply a medium-sized spread of but butter on top of your pancakes

- Place your banana slices on top, followed by the maple syrup

Chia Seed and Almond Butter Pudding

Ingredients:

- Cleaned chia seeds

- Fresh almond milk

- Almond butter

- Blueberries or strawberries

- Optional: honey

Directions:

- Make a mixture of almond milk and chia seeds, and place in the fridge overnight

- In the morning, top up your mixture with fresh berries and almond butter

- If preferred, drizzle with honey

Lunch Meals

Quinoa With Chickpea Salad

Ingredients:

- Well-cooked quinoa

- Chickpeas, drained and rinsed

- Diced cucumber

- Cherry tomatoes, cut into halves

- Optional: feta cheese

- Dressing (lemon tahini)

Instructions:

- Combine chickpeas, cucumber, quinoa, and tomatoes in a mixing bowl

- Add in feta cheese, if desired

- Drizzle the lemon tahini dressing on top

The Grilled Salmon Fish With Avocado Wrap

Ingredients:

- Tortilla or full-grain wrap

- Grilled salmon filet

- Sliced avocado

- Greens (mixed)

- Greek Yogurt (dill sauce)

Directions:

- Lay your wrap down and nicely place the grilled salmon, mixed greens, and avocado, and drizzle the dill sauce

- Then, roll it up and enjoy your meal

The Mediterranean Chickpea Bowl

Ingredients:

- Cooked brown rice or quinoa

- Well-roasted spiced chickpeas in olive oil

- Washed spinach leaves

- Cherry tomatoes, cut in halves

- Kalamata olives

- Feta cheese

Directions:

- In a mixing bowl, combine the tomatoes, roasted chickpeas, quinoa, feta cheese, and olives

Caprese-Stuffed Avocado

Ingredients:

- Avocado, fresh and soft

- Fresh mozzarella cheese, sliced

- Halved cherry tomatoes

- Basil leaves

- Balsamic glaze

Directions:

- Create a well in the avocado by scooping out the middle of the avocado

- Place the tomatoes, mozzarella cheese slices, and your fresh basil leaves inside the well

- Drizzle with Balsamic glaze

Fresh Vegetable Stir-Fry and Asian-Inspired Tofu

Ingredients:

- Cubed, firm tofu

- Freshly mixed vegetables (snap peas, broccoli, bell peppers)

- Quinoa or brown rice

- Soy sauce

- Minced garlic and ginger

- Sesame oil

Directions:

- In a pan, use your sesame oil to saute vegetables and tofu with garlic and ginger

- Serve on top of quinoa or brown rice, with a drizzle of soy sauce

Dinner Meals

Sweet Potato and Grilled Chicken With Asparagus

Ingredients:

- Grilled chicken breast

- Roasted sweet potato

- Grilled asparagus

- Herbs with olive oil, if preferred

Directions:

- Grill your seasoned chicken

- Grill your asparagus and roast the sweet potatoes

Turkey Meatballs and Spaghetti Squash

Ingredients:

- Shredded and roasted spaghetti squash

- Fat-free turkey meatballs

- Sugar-free tomato sauce

- Parmesan cheese

- Washed fresh basil

Directions:

- Top up your spaghetti squash with the turkey meatballs and tomato sauce

- Sprinkle the Parmesan cheese on top

- Use the basil to garnish the dish

Vegetable Curry With Lentils

Ingredients:

- Lentils (cooked)

- Mixed vegetables, such as cauliflower, carrots, and peas

- Fresh coconut milk

- Curry spices, such as coriander, cumin, and turmeric

- Basmati rice

Directions:

- In a coconut milk sauce, simmer your cooked lentils

- Serve it on top of the basmati rice

Quinoa With Baked Cod and Steamed Broccoli

Ingredients:

- Baked cod filet, sauced with lemon juice and herbs

- Quinoa, cooked

- Fresh broccoli florets, steamed

- Optional: lemon butter sauce

Directions:

- Make a bed of quinoa on a dinner plate

- Place the baked quinoa and steamed broccoli

- Drizzle it with lemon-butter sauce, if preferred

Quinoa and Black beans With Stuffed Bell Peppers

Ingredients:

- Halved and seeded bell peppers

- Black beans, cooked

- Quinoa, cooked

- Tomatoes, diced

- Optional: Cheddar cheese

Directions:

- Make a mixture of quinoa, black beans and tomatoes (diced) and stuff with the bell pepper

- Bake it, topped up with cheese, until it is heated all the way through

Snacks

Berry Parfait With Greek Yogurt

Ingredients:

- Yogurt (Greek)

- Mixture of berries

- Low-sugar granola

Directions:

- Arrange berries, granola, and Greek yogurt in a glass for a great testing parfait

Veggie Platter and Hummus

Ingredients:

- Homemade hummus, or you can use a store-bought brand

- Different types of vegetables, such as cucumbers, bell pepper strips, and carrots

Directions:

- Place and arrange your veggies inside the bowl with hummus

Dried Fruits With Mixed Nuts

Ingredients:

- Various types of nuts, such as cashews, almonds, and walnuts.

- Dried fruits, such as cranberries, figs, and apricots

Directions:

- Combine all the ingredients to get a well-balanced and satisfying meal plan

References

Carroll, C. (2021, June 28). *Is the Mediterranean diet a healthier way for you to eat?* Verywell Fit. https://www.verywellfit.com/the-mediterranean-diet-pros-and-cons-4685664

Davidson, C. (2017, January 3). *Beginner's guide to a plant-based diet.* Forks over Knives. https://www.forksoverknives.com/how-tos/plant-based-primer-beginners-guide-starting-plant-based-diet/

Dr. Sears Zone. (n.d.). *What is the zone diet? Learn what it means to be in the zone.* Zone Living. https://zoneliving.com/pages/zone-diet

Good Food Is Good Medicine. (2022, February 4). *Intermittent fasting: Benefits, how it works, and is it right for you?* Good-Food. https://health.ucdavis.edu/blog/good-food/intermittent-fasting-benefits-how-it-works-and-is-it-right-for-you/2022/02#:~:text=How%20does%20intermittent%20fasting%20work

Goodreads. (n.d.-a). *Marla Heller quotes (author of the dash diet weight loss solution).* Goodreads. https://www.goodreads.com/author/quotes/240198.Marla_Heller

Goodreads. (n.d.-b). *Paleo quotes (15 quotes).* Goodreads. https://www.goodreads.com/quotes/tag/paleo#:~:text=Food%20is%20celebratory%2C%20nourishing.

Goodreads (n.d.). *Barry Sears quotes (author of The Zone).* Goodreads https://www.goodreads.com/author/quotes/148120.Barry_Sears

Juma, N. (2023, May 21). *Keto quotes for the low-carb lifestyle*. Everyday Power. https://everydaypower.com/keto-quotes/

Maricic, D. (2023, September 6). *Let's eat in a Mediterranean way - 20 inspirational quotes*. Archi-Living. https://www.archi-living.com/53399/lets-eat-in-a-mediterranean-way-20-inspirational-quotes/

McAllister, M. (2022, April 1). *21 quotes on intermittent fasting*. Melissa Made Online. https://www.google.com/amp/s/melissamadeonline.com/2022/04/01/21-quotes-on-intermittent-fasting/amp/

McNamara, A. (n.d.). *75 best food quotes and captions*. Toast. https://pos.toasttab.com/blog/on-the-line/food-quotes-and-captions

NHLBI. (2021). *The science behind the DASH eating plan*. National Heart, Lung, and Blood Institute. https://www.nhlbi.nih.gov/education/dash/research#:~:text=The%20results%20of%20these%20studies

Shoemaker, S. (2022, May 27). *Weight watchers diet review: Does it work for weight loss?* Healthline. https://www.healthline.com/nutrition/weight-watchers-diet-review#TOC_TITLE_HDR_1

Streit, L. (2022, January 14). *The flexitarian diet: A detailed beginner's guide*. Healthline. https://www.healthline.com/nutrition/flexitarian-diet-guide

The Flexitarian Rx Quotes. (2023, October 10). *Quotes*. The Flexitarian Rx. https://theflexitarianrx.com/category/quotes/

The Paleo Diet. (2020, February 4). *The benefits of the paleo diet*. The Paleo Diet. https://thepaleodiet.com/benefits-of-the-paleo-diet/

www.ingramcontent.com/pod-product-compliance
Lightning Source LLC
Chambersburg PA
CBHW050732260726

48661CB00001B/188